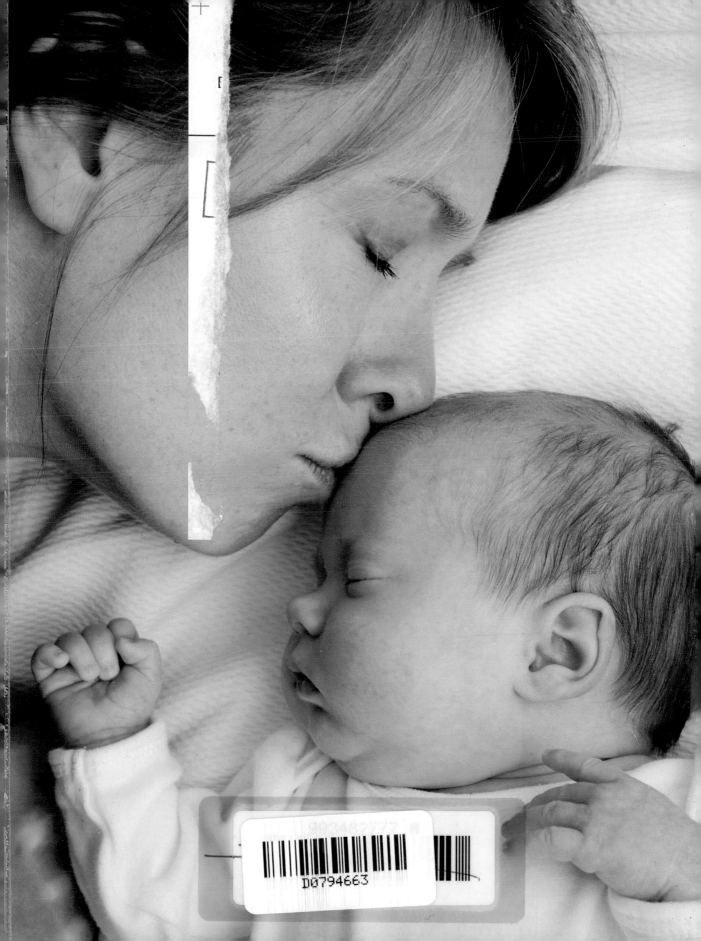

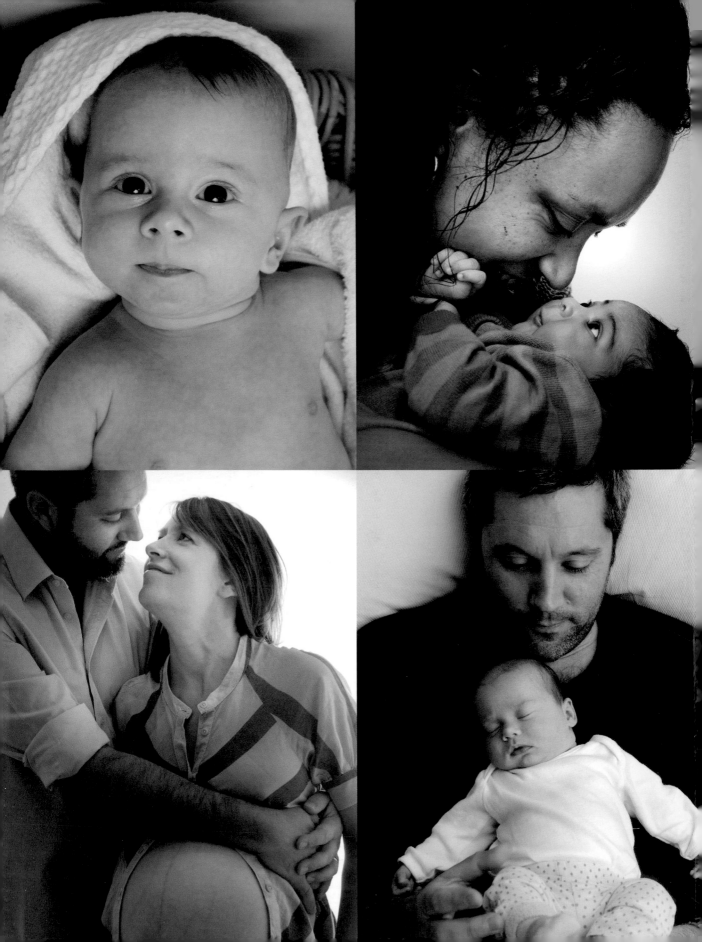

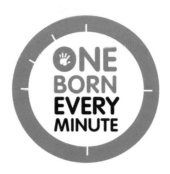

Your Pregnancy

Week
by
Week

Midwife Vickie Hugo

Quadrille
PUBLISHING

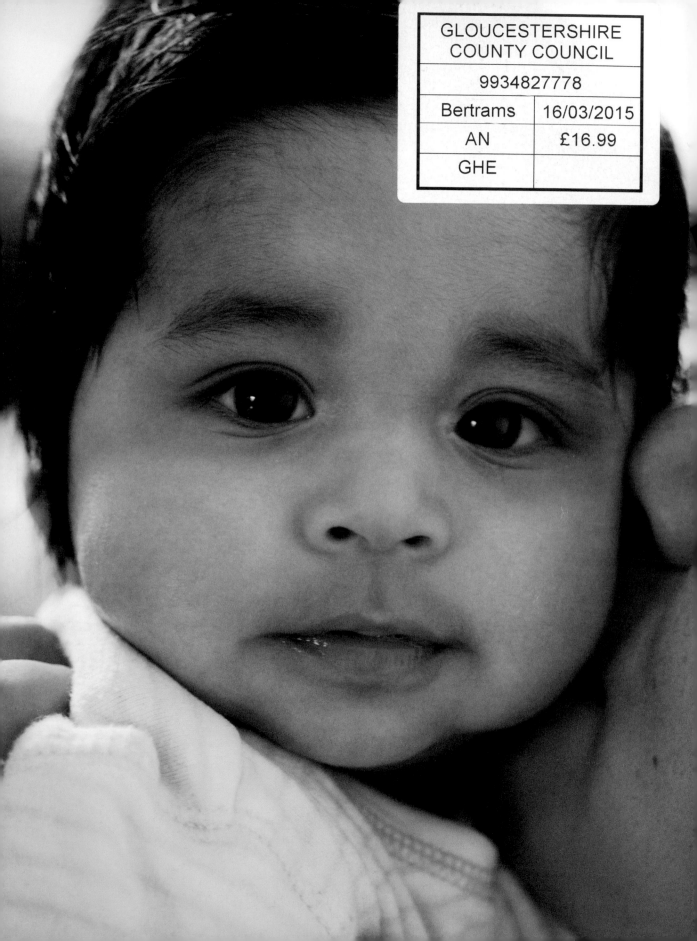

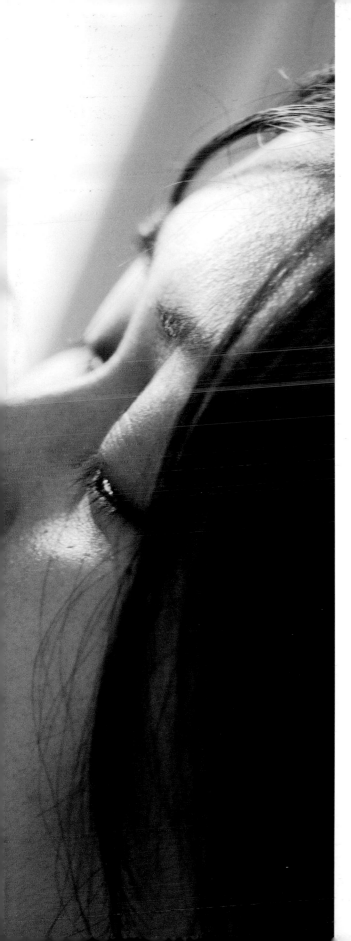

Contents

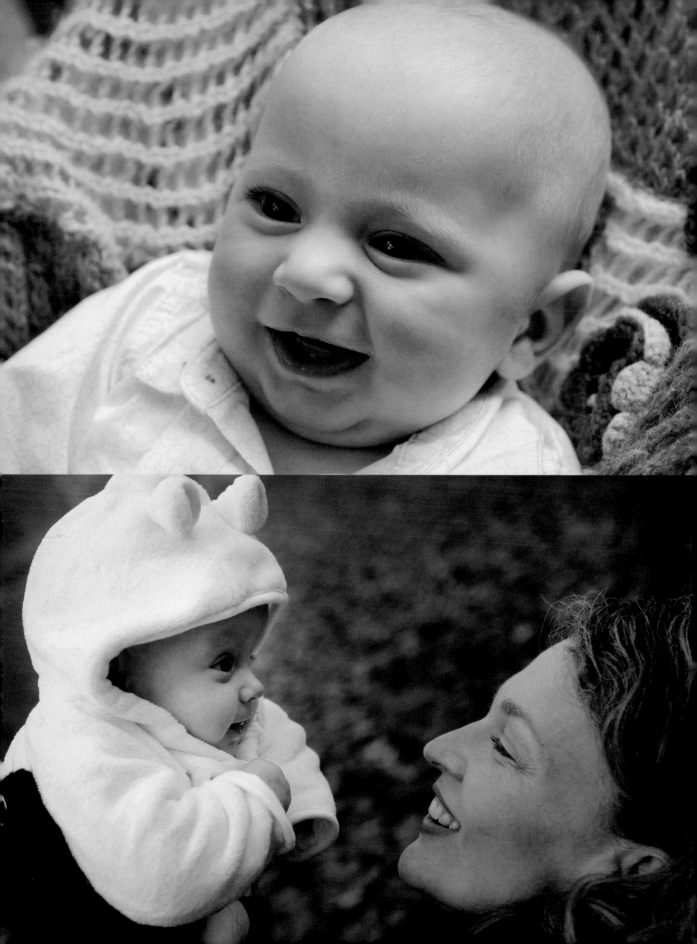

Introduction

Despite having studied and practised midwifery for more than ten years, I am still completely amazed by the miracle of childbirth. It must be the single most life-changing event a family can go through, and it is an absolute privilege to witness and be a part of this on a daily basis.

Pregnancy and birth are unique to each individual. Many different factors will influence people's thoughts and feelings, and many different variables will affect labour and birth. It can be overwhelming to expect your first and your subsequent babies with so many things to consider and prepare for before that new baby arrives in the world. I am hoping that this book provides a useful guide in staying informed about the choices available to you: staying healthy, helping you to prepare for birth and motherhood, learning what is happening week by week, and knowing what the options are during labour and delivery.

I hope it goes a long way in explaining a baffling world where art, science and culture meet, and where safety is the main objective in achieving the world's most basic yet most celebrated event. New life.

Vickie Hugo
Midwife

You are pregnant!

Congratulations! Discovering you are pregnant can be one of the most joyful moments of your life. It's important to be practical and let your healthcare professionals know you are pregnant so that your antenatal care can begin. They will monitor your baby's progress throughout pregnancy and provide you with medical care and advice. Finding out about the healthcare and birthing options available in your area will allow you to make choices that are right for you.

What Happens Now?

Step one is to let your doctor know you are pregnant, so book an appointment with your GP as soon as you find out. He or she will start the ball rolling with your antenatal care.

Your GP visit

Most women are 4–8 weeks pregnant when they take a pregnancy test. If that is the case with you, contact your GP without delay. This way you will be in the system in time for the option of screening test that are carried out between 12 and 13 weeks for abnormalities.

Your GP will ask you when the first day of your last period was, to work out your estimated due date (EDD). An ultrasound scan later on (see page 43) will establish a more accurate due date, so your healthcare providers can know roughly when you conceived and check your baby is doing well for his or her 'gestational age' (the time since conception). Your GP surgery will arrange your booking appointment with a midwife.

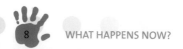

Antenatal care

Antenatal care varies from one area to the next and also depends on whether you choose to have a hospital birth or a home birth.

Shared care

If you want to give birth in hospital, your care may be shared between your GP and the community midwives based at your surgery or a health centre. If you have a medical condition or complications in your pregnancy, you'll also see the obstetric team and midwives at the hospital. Your antenatal appointments will be run by your community midwife and you'll go to the hospital for ultrasound scans and blood tests. During labour, you'll be attended by a hospital midwife. A community midwife, then a health visitor will visit you when you're back home.

Team midwifery

In team midwifery, a team of midwives (based at a hospital or GP's surgery) looks after a number of women during pregnancy and labour. If you are allocated to a team of midwives, you will have a main midwife, but will also see others in the team if your midwife is unavailable.

Who's who in antenatal care?

Midwives

These professionals are trained to care for women who have a normal pregnancy and birth. They work with obstetricians and ask for their advanced medical expertise when necessary. Midwives run antenatal appointments and talk expectant mothers through test results. They work as either hospital or community midwives. Hospital midwives work on the antenatal wards and delivery suites, looking after women in labour, delivering their babies and on the postnatal wards . Community midwives are based at GP surgeries, children's centres or hospitals, and assist women through home births, hospital births (if in a team) or births at midwifery units or birth centres.

Obstetricians

These doctors are trained in the care of pregnant women. They work in hospitals alongside midwives. It's unlikely that you'll see an obstetrician unless you're over 40, have a medical condition, became pregnant using assisted conception, have had an operation in the abdominal area or are obese. If a complication arises during pregnancy, your midwife will consult with an obstetrician to make sure you receive the right care. If you need a Caesarean section or other assisted delivery (see pages 122–130), an obstetrician will perform the procedures.

Your Birth Options

Your GP and/or midwife will want to know where you wish to give birth – at home, in the hospital or at a birth centre. Choices vary depending on if your pregnancy is low or high risk, and what your local authority can offer you. Find out what's available in your area to make the right decision for you and your baby.

Making a choice

You'll be asked early in pregnancy where you want to give birth. You don't have to stick to any decision you make now; later on, you may feel differently. It's easy to become overwhelmed when faced with unfamiliar choices. The information below gives you the lay of the land. It's important to keep an open mind, as labour is unpredictable. For instance, you may want a home birth, but if a medical complication arises it may be best to transfer to the hospital for the safety and of you of your baby.

Hospital birth

Most women in the UK opt for a hospital birth. Many women like knowing that, should a complication arise, medical staff are right there. (Statistically, complications arise more in first labours.) If you live far from a hospital (making it hard to get there during a home birth, should you need to), or if you've had complications in a previous birth, you might feel more confident giving birth in hospital. Also, many women prefer to give birth at a hospital because of the range of pain-relief options available.

Obstetricians and midwives tend to advise women to give birth at a hospital if they have previously had a Caesarean section, are over 40, are obese or have a medical condition. If antenatal test results suggest that your baby may need medical assistance , it is wise to give birth at a hospital so that your baby will immediately receive the help he needs.

There are three types of maternity unit within hospitals in the UK:
✦ obstetric unit (OU): this is a hospital department in which midwives, obstetricians and anaesthetists work together, so an obstetrician, neonatal unit and the full range of pain-relief medications are available. Most births take place in an OU, where there is minimum risk and maximum facilities

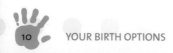

✦ alongside midwifery unit (AMU): sometimes called a birth centre, this may be part of an OU or is run alongside one. An AMU is staffed by midwives and offers a limited range of pain-relief options. It is close to the OU for easy access to obstetricians and a neonatal unit, if necessary
✦ freestanding midwifery unit (FMU): also called a birth centre, this type of unit is affiliated with a hospital and is staffed by midwives. It offers a limited range of pain-relief options. If obstetric or neonatal facilities are needed, you would be transferred to hospital by ambulance.

Find out which facilities are available in your area. Contact the OUs, AMUs and FMUs to find out when they organise tours of their units. Feel free to ask the staff any questions you may have. Also, ask mothers in your area who have recently given birth how they rate the facilities they used. Bear in mind that each woman has a unique birth experience, and you may well feel comfortable in a situation that isn't right for another woman. Gather as much information as you can before you make a decision.

Home birth

If this is your second or subsequent birth, your previous pregnancies were normal, you've had a normal vaginal delivery in the past and this pregnancy is progressing normally, a home birth is a low-risk option for you. If this is your first baby, it's a less risky option if you are under 40, not obese, in good health, your pregnancy is progressing normally and you live near a hospital, should a quick transfer become necessary.

There are advantages to a home birth. If hospitals make you anxious, the idea of giving birth at home may be comforting. You can involve more people than just your birth partners. Also, you can ensure that any equipment you want to use (say, a birthing pool) is there for you (it might not be available in the hospital). You don't have to get to hospital while in labour. It's likely that the midwives who come to your home will be the same as those who cared for you during pregnancy, as a team of community midwives usually deals with home births (see page 9). Also, you won't be separated from your partner at any time during the process.

Home births are rising in popularity, and recent studies confirm that they are no more of a risk than hospital births in cases where the mother has had a previous normal vaginal delivery. For first-time births, the risks of complications arising are three times higher than for those who have had a previous birth, but the actual number of negative outcomes is very low. If you want a home birth, ask your midwife or GP if there is any medical or practical reason for it is inadvisable for you to choose this option.

Eating Healthily

Eating a balanced, varied diet packed with nutritious foods will maximize your baby's chances for a healthy life and also improve your experience of pregnancy, birth and those challenging first few weeks after the delivery.

Iron

This mineral is vital to the development of your baby's bones and muscles, and to your own good health. You need two or three times as much iron in your diet when you are pregnant, so eat more foods that are rich sources, such as meat, fish and eggs. It's easier to absorb iron from red meat than from other sources of iron. Vitamin C can help your body to absorb more iron from the food you eat, so try drinking a glass of orange juice with a meal. Tea and coffee, on the other hand, make it harder for your body to extract iron from foods. Avoid drinking these around mealtimes.

If your body lacks iron, you are at risk of developing anaemia during pregnancy (see page 73). If you think you may have become anaemic, speak to your midwife or GP, who can prescribe an iron supplement. Don't take an iron supplement without your midwife's or GP's guidance, as unnecessary iron supplements can damage the heart and liver.

A varied diet

Variety is the key to a balanced diet, which should contain proteins, fats, carbohydrates, fibre, vitamins and minerals from a wide range of sources. Try to eat something every day from each of the food groups listed below.

Meat, fish, pulses, beans and nuts

These foods provide the body with proteins, which are vital for the healthy development of your baby's bones, muscles and internal organs, and help your own body to create and repair cells. Roughly one-third of each meal should consist of a protein element. Animal sources of protein (such as lean meats, fish, dairy products and well-cooked eggs) and soya products contain all the types of proteins we need. If you are a vegetarian or a vegan, you'll need a variety of vegetable sources to meet your body's protein requirements (see below).

Bread, cereals, potatoes, pasta and rice

These carbohydrates fuel your body, giving it the energy needed to support the baby's development and continue with your day-to-day tasks. The main part of each meal should consist of the carbohydrate element. Choose wholegrain (or unrefined) carbohydrates, such as wholemeal flour or pasta, brown bread or brown rice. These have more vitamins, minerals and fibre than the white (or refined) versions.

Fruits and vegetables

Fresh, frozen and dried fruits and vegetables are full of vitamins and minerals. They also contain fibre, which helps to prevent and alleviate constipation, a common side effect of pregnancy. Eating a wide variety of fruits and vegetables supplies your body with a range of vitamins and minerals. Limit your intake of fruit juice, which has a high sugar content. Eating too much sugar in pregnancy increases your chances of developing gestational diabetes, which can be dangerous to both you and the baby.

Dairy products

Milk, cheese, yogurt and cream provide calcium, which is necessary for your baby's developing bones and muscles. They are also sources of vitamins A, B and D. It's worth remembering that the lower the fat content of dairy products, the easier they are to digest and the more nutrients they contain. If you do not take in enough calcium during pregnancy, your body will draw on your body's own reserves of it for the baby, which could cause osteoporosis in later life, so make sure you eat plenty of calcium during pregnancy.

Vitamin supplements

Take folic acid and vitamin D supplements during pregnancy as it is difficult to obtain enough of these nutrients from your food. You need a 400mcg dose of folic acid each day in order to prevent spina bifida and other neural tube defects in the baby (or a higher dosage, if you have had a baby with spina bifida or if you are obese). Ideally, you should begin to take folic acid three months before you become pregnant (so if you are trying for a baby, start taking it now) and continue to take it until the end of the first trimester. You also need a 10mg dose of vitamin D each day, which you should take right the way through pregnancy and until you stop breastfeeding. This will help to prevent osteoporosis in later life.

Changing your diet

Many women begin to think more carefully about their diet when they become pregnant, and your pregnancy can provide a fantastic motivation for you, your partner and any children you already have to improve the way you all eat. Eating healthily as a family means that you can encourage one another and work together to come up with ideas for wholesome meals and snacks. It also means that you can each help one another to stick to the healthier way of eating.

If you would like improve your diet, the key to success is to make changes slowly, rather than starting an all-new regime overnight. Plunging headlong into new, healthier eating patters makes it difficult

Vegetarian/ Vegan Diet

It is challenging for vegetarians and vegans to obtain calcium, vitamin D, vitamin B12 (which is found only in animal products, so take supplements if you are a vegan) and iron (a lack of which can cause anaemia – see box, opposite). If you eat dairy products and fish as part of a varied diet, your body will probably take in enough of these essential nutrients to stay healthy and support your baby's development. If you are a vegan, make sure you eat more pulses, tofu, leafy green vegetables, wholegrain foods and nuts to maximize your intake of essential nutrients and proteins. Ask your midwife or GP for advice if you have any concerns.

to resist temptation when your work colleagues open a packet of biscuits. It's difficult to change all your undesirable eating habits in one go; instead, make one change at a time. And allow yourself to fall off the wagon occasionally – just make sure that it isn't too often.

Reducing sugar

One of the best ways to improve your diet is to reduce the amount of refined sugar you eat. Sugar sneaks into our diets to the point that many people consume far more than is healthy. Many foods that contain refined sugar have little nutritional value. While they may give you an initial burst of energy, you are likely to feel a dip in energy soon afterwards, and then begin to crave more sugar. In this way, sugar is highly addictive.

Biscuits, chocolate, cakes and sweets, fizzy drinks, cereal bars, breakfast bars and many breakfast cereals are all chock-full of sugar. Breakfast cereals are among the worst culprits, even those that are advertised as 'healthy' – many are very high in sugar (ie, they contain more than 12.5g sugar per 100g). It is definitely worth reading the labels to ensure, before buying, that you pick a healthier one.

Too much sugar in the diet can lead to high blood pressure and diabetes, and becoming overweight or obese (see box on page 16).

Try immediately to reduce the amount of sugar you eat. Remove all sugary snacks from the house. If you take sugar in tea and coffee, leave it out (it won't take long before you don't notice the difference). Instead of snacking on biscuits and other sweet treats, munch on healthy snacks (see page 16 for a list of suggestions). Buy breakfast cereals that have a low amount of added sugar, and use fruit (strawberries and bananas are good) to sweeten your cereal instead. Take healthy snacks to work to help you resist the sugary snacks filled with 'empty' calories that your workmates share with one another.

Planning your meals

It is much easier to stick to a healthy diet if you plan and shop for your meals in advance. Sit down with your partner and decide between you which meals you would like to eat over the course of a week. Write a list of all the ingredients you need, and shop for those things only. This way you don't end up buying a bunch of unnecessary things on a whim. If you avoid food shopping on an empty stomach, it's easier to walk past the aisles containing confectionery and high-calorie/low-nutrition snacks without picking up that naughty treat.

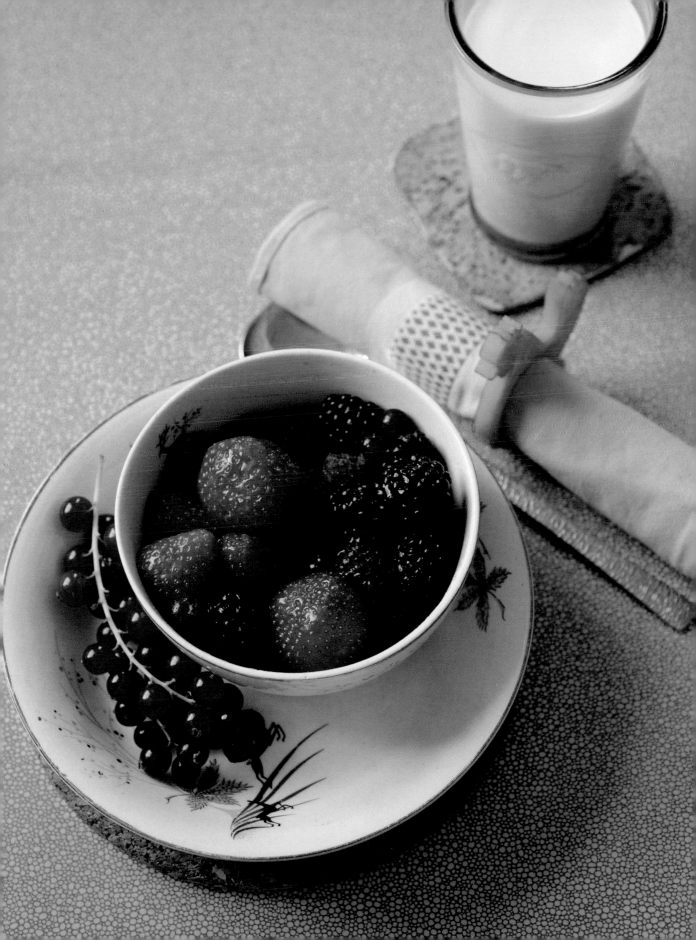

Weight gain and obesity

A woman with a healthy BMI (body mass index) should gain roughly 13kg during pregnancy. Only 1kg of this is gained during the first trimester. In the second and third trimesters, weight gain is at 500–700g per week. Much of this weight gain is accounted for by the baby herself, the placenta, the amniotic fluid, the increased amount of blood in the body, water retention and the increased size of your breasts and womb. You don't need to consume any extra calories during the first and second trimesters; stick to the recommended amount of 2,000 calories per day for a healthy woman. In the third trimester, though, you will need to eat 200–300 extra calories per day.

If you are obese, you should aim not to put on any weight during pregnancy. Use the support of your GP or midwife to help you, and ask family and friends to consider eating a healthy diet alongside as encouragement. Your GP or midwife will monitor your health and that of your baby regularly, as being obese brings an increased risk of pregnancy complications such as high blood pressure, gestational diabetes and pre-eclampsia. There is greater risk of stillbirth, the need for medical interventions during birth and postpartum hemorrhage.

Do some research and look into how to make the meals you usually cook more nutritious. You could throw some beans into a stew or a casserole, add lentils to soups and toasted seeds to salads, switch to wholemeal pasta and brown rice and cook (preferably by steaming) a second vegetable with your meals. There are many books to choose from, and many supermarkets offer menu cards with healthy ideas for meals to help out busy mums. A little research and planning will go a long way.

Eating at work

Planning for and taking your lunches to work can provide a double bonus. Not only will you save a fortune on buying prepared lunches but you will also avoid all the high-fat, high-sugar options. Taking in leftovers (simply cook extra to take in the next day) is the easiest and quickest way of ensuring you have a good meal at lunchtime. Alternatively, plan your lunches and shop for them. Take healthy snacks (see below) to see you through the mid-morning and mid-afternoon dips.

Healthy snacks

Snacks are often where people fall down when trying to eat healthily. It's too easy to open a packet of crisps or biscuits when you need a little pick-me-up and you're too busy to think about what to have or prepare something nutritious. Healthy snacking does require a little thought and effort, but once you're into the swing of it, it simply becomes habit like anything else.

Try the following suggestions:
✦ dried fruit, such as apricots, raisins, apples and bananas
✦ fresh fruits such as apples, oranges and berries
✦ unsalted nuts and seeds
✦ oatcakes, with or without cheese
✦ natural yogurt (sweeten it with fruit or honey)
✦ pasta salad (made with wholemeal pasta)
✦ cold skinless chicken breast in a brown wrap or roll
✦ hummus with chopped vegetables such as cucumber, carrots and peppers.

Eating out/takeaways

There's nothing wrong with the odd treat, and eating out – or grabbing a takeaway when you're too tired to cook – can be good for the soul!

When eating in a restaurant, try to choose one of the healthier options from the menu. Avoid rich sauces and deep-fried items. Also, many restaurants provide enormous portions, so don't feel as if you have to polish off the plate – use your brain rather than your tummy to decide when you have eaten enough.

Takeaways tend to be greasy and full of fat, and it can be hard to make a healthy selection. So keep these as occasional treats, and try to make sure you limit eating other treats around a takeaway to make up for it!

Foods to avoid

Pregnant women should avoid eating certain foods that pose risks to the baby. Keep the following foods out of your diet until after the baby is born:
+ liver and liver products
+ raw or undercooked eggs
+ raw or undercooked meat
+ unpasteurised and blue cheeses
+ pâtés
+ bagged salads.

In addition to this, do not store cooked meats such as ham for more than a few days, and ensure that they are kept in hygienic conditions. Also, care should be taken with seafood. Although fish is highly nutritious, certain types should be limited during pregnancy or avoided completely. Swordfish, shark and marlin tend to contain high mercury levels and should not be eaten during pregnancy. Limit oily fish, such as salmon, fresh tuna and mackerel, to no more than two portions per week. You can eat tinned tuna more frequently. Raw seafood and shellfish carry a higher risk of food poisoning and parasitic infections, but they are safe to eat if thoroughly cooked. Raw fish that has been previously frozen is fine, as the freezing process kills off any parasites.

Kitchen hygiene

A little extra care and attention are required when it comes to hygiene in the kitchen because pregnant women are more likely to get gastroenteritis, caused by bacteria and viruses. The chances of complications arising from such infections are also increased for pregnant women.

The following tips will help you to reduce your chances of infection:
+ wash your hands before and after handling food
+ wash all fruits and vegetables very well and scrub them when necessary
+ wash kitchen utensils and knives in very hot water using detergent, and rinse and dry them well
+ use dedicated knives, utensils and chopping boards for different types of ingredients – keep chopping boards and knives especially for raw meat and fish, and always use a separate board and knife for vegetables
+ wash and change tea towels, hand towels and dishcloths regularly
+ ensure frozen foods are thoroughly defrosted before cooking
+ reheat food until it is piping hot, be especially careful when using a microwave oven that the food is heated all the way through, and never reheat food more than once
+ if you are unsure how long an item of food has been stored in the freezer, throw it away.

Keeping Active

It is perfectly safe to exercise during pregnancy. In fact, staying fit and strong will make it easier for your body to deal with pregnancy, labour and the challenging first few weeks of your baby's life outside the womb.

Be careful!

Make sure that you eat a while before and after you exercise, drink plenty of water to keep well hydrated, and don't allow yourself to become overheated. If you find it difficult to breathe or become light-headed, develop a headache, feel any pain during exercise (particularly abdominal or lower back pain) or experience chest pains or palpitations, see your GP or midwife.

Exercises for pregnancy

There are many good reasons for getting some exercise when you are pregnant. Besides being great for lifting the mood and good for heart health, exercise can help you to overcome many of the side effects of pregnancy, such as varicose veins, tiredness and insomnia. Being strong and well toned can help you to deliver your baby more easily, too.

Low-impact exercises that increase the heart rate within safe limits, don't allow you to become too dehydrated and increase muscle tone without stretching ligaments and abdominal muscles too much are the most appropriate for pregnancy. Swimming, cycling, gentle gym classes such as yoga and Pilates (ideally, classes for pregnant women), and brisk walking are ideal. Aim to raise your heartbeat slightly and become out of breath.

Avoid exercises that put too much strain on your joints, back or womb. If you like to lift weights, begin using lighter weights to avoid permanently damaging your joints, ligaments and tendons. Due to pregnancy hormones these are all looser than normal and prone to damage.

Certain sports should be avoided, such as those in which you could fall (e.g. horse riding or skiing), contact sports (e.g. football or judo), jogging or running (or any exercise that requires jumping), sports performed at a high altitude, scuba diving, or any exercise in which you lay on your back.

If you already have a fitness regime, it's likely that you'll continue with it during pregnancy – although it's worth considering whether or not you need to change it to make it more appropriate for pregnancy. If you don't make a habit of regular exercise, your body won't be used to it, so take up something gentle, such as yoga, Pilates, cycling or swimming.

It's important that you listen to your body and pace yourself. Don't overdo it, and rest when you feel you need to.

Pelvic-floor exercises

You've probably heard of pelvic-floor exercises and may have practised them already, but exercising your pelvic-floor muscles is even more important during pregnancy. This is because the weight of the growing baby in the womb during pregnancy puts great strain on these muscles, as does the birth itself. Once they are stretched and damaged by pregnancy and birth, they cannot provide adequate support for the womb, bladder, vagina, rectum and bowels, leading to stress incontinence (see page 91) in the short and long term. Strong pelvic-floor muscles will make it less likely that you will experience these problems after birth or in the long term. And they can enhance your sex life, too!

To exercise the pelvic-floor muscles (around the anus, vagina and urethra), you squeeze the muscles as you do when you need to stop yourself urinating. You won't be able to see any movement, but the pelvic-floor area will feel as if it is lifting when you squeeze.

There are two types of pelvic-floor exercises that you should do:

✦ make slow squeezes, holding each squeeze for a count of ten (build up to ten if you find it difficult at first). Repeat ten times. Make sure that you are breathing normally while you squeeze and hold

✦ make quick squeezes, releasing and squeezing to a count of ten without holding the squeezes.

Once you can manage slow squeezes to a count of ten, increase the hold to a count of fifteen. When ten quick squeezes in a row become easy, increase it to fifteen. This way, you will continue to strengthen the muscles.

Try to exercise at the same time each day. Use a reminder – say, each time you stop at a traffic light, or when you relax to watch television in the evening, when you take a shower or when you first get into bed – so that you remember to practise them regularly.

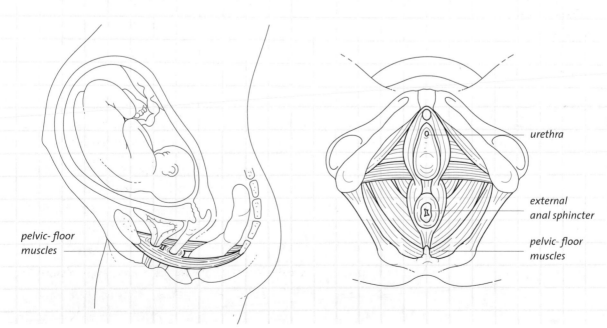

pelvic-floor muscles

urethra

external anal sphincter

pelvic-floor muscles

Your General Health

Taking care of your health has never been more important and you need to limit your exposure to certain things that could harm your baby. There are many scare stories about what does and doesn't harm a baby during pregnancy. Don't let them alarm you. Focus on the following advice, which is scientifically proven and reliable.

Substances to avoid

It is widely known that drinking alcohol, smoking cigarettes and taking recreational drugs during pregnancy are all harmful to the unborn baby. But do you know how they are harmful?

Alcohol

Regular excessive drinking greatly increases the risk of developing complications in your pregnancy and harming your baby. The odd glass of wine now and then won't do any damage, but consuming a large amount of alcohol in one go should be avoided. Many women are completely put off alcohol during the morning-sickness stage, and continue to abstain altogether or cut down until after pregnancy. If you had a heavy night of drinking before you realised you were pregnant, don't worry. It's unlikely that one night will have caused harm to your baby – but don't do it again!

Cigarettes

Smoking cigarettes and other tobacco products affects the supply of both oxygen and nutrients to your unborn baby, and also increases the risk of miscarriage and other pregnancy complications. You are also more likely to have a premature baby or low-birthweight baby if you smoke. Passive smoking also carries these risks.

Recreational drugs

If you take cocaine, cannabis, heroin or amphetamines, they will enter the baby's bloodstream and potentially cause damage. Cocaine and ecstasy are known to cause placental bleeding and intracranial bleeding in the fetus or neonate. In addition, recreational drugs are linked to premature labour and low-birthweight babies. Habitual drug use will cause the baby to be born with withdrawal symptoms, for which she will require help.

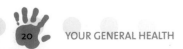

Caffeine

It's a good idea to reduce your caffeine intake during pregnancy because caffeine dehydrates the body and reduces the amount of calcium, iron and vitamin C that the body absorbs from food. Like many pregnant women, you may find you don't want to drink as much coffee or other caffeinated drinks, especially while you suffer from morning sickness. You may therefore be quite happy to reduce caffeinated drinks or cut them out altogether during your pregnancy.

Environmental factors

Some chemicals can have a harmful effect on a developing baby, especially during the early few weeks of pregnancy. What is and isn't harmful can be confusing, as misinformation abounds. Bear in mind the following:

Harmful

You'll need to limit your exposure to industrial chemicals such as solvents, paints, lacquers and cleaning agents if you work in a dry-cleaner's shop, garage, laboratory, in certain factories or as an artist. Ensure your workspace is well ventilated and that your clothing is suitably protective.

Not harmful

Hair dyes have not been found to be harmful if used in normal amounts. Neither has exposure to office equipment such as computers, printers or photocopiers. Microwave ovens are safe to use.

The chemicals found in ordinary household cleaning and decorating products have not been proven to harm unborn babies, but it makes good sense not to inhale the fumes from cleaning products, glue, paint or petrol. (A word of warning: if you need to strip paint and you are not sure whether or not the paint is leadfree, get someone else to strip it because, even in small amounts, lead could harm the baby.)

Radiation from X-rays is harmful only in large quantities. Unless you have had a large number of X-rays in the abdominal area before you were eight weeks pregnant, your baby will not be harmed. As a precaution, however, doctors will avoid giving you an X-ray if they know you are pregnant.

There have been reports that ultrasound scanners can cause problems that are linked with leukaemia in developing babies, but these have now been disproven.

Getting help for addiction

If you find it difficult to cut down on your alcohol intake during pregnancy, or stop smoking or using drugs, speak to your GP or midwife. There are specialist midwives who are very knowlegeable about drugs and addiction and will not judge you. They can support you in stopping or reducing your intake safely.

Medicines

Although it's wise to avoid taking any medication during pregnancy if possible (as medications are not tested on pregnant women), some over-the-counter and prescribed medicines are known to be harmful to developing babies, while others are unlikely to harm a developing fetus.

Over-the-counter medications

If you need to take a painkiller during pregnancy, stick to paracetamol. Do not take ibuprofen or codeine, and avoid aspirin, too, unless it is prescribed for high blood pressure, obesity or previous recurrent miscarriage. Antihistamines are considered safe to use in pregnancy, but avoid cold and flu remedies (use paracetamol combined with a hot lemon drink instead). Diuretics (to control fluid retention) should be avoided. This is because, while fluid retention (oedema) is common during pregnancy (see page 66), it is also a symptom of pre-eclampsia, a dangerous condition that can arise in pregnant women. Using a diuretic could hide this telling symptom. If you experience any sudden swelling in the hands, feet or legs, speak to your GP or midwife without delay.

Prescription/hospital/vaccinations/travel drugs

Some most commonly used antibiotics are safe to use during pregnancy, including amoxicillin, ampicillin, penicillin, erythromycin and clindamycin. Avoid using antibiotics from the tetracycline family.

Any surgery is usually postponed until after the pregnancy. If you do need emergency surgery during your pregnancy, it's possible that it will be performed under regional or local anaesthetic. There is no clinical evidence to suggest that anaesthetics will harm a developing baby.

If your GP's surgery offers you a flu jab, it's a good idea to take. The same applies for the whooping cough jab, which will be offered to you between 28 and 38 weeks. Both vaccinations will provide your baby with protection after he is born. In some cases, you can have these two vaccinations at the same time.

Many pregnant women take a holiday before the baby arrives, while it is still safe to travel. If you need to be vaccinated, cholera, tetanus and polio vaccines are safe during pregnancy. Consult the Department of Health's website for information on the safety of other travel vaccines. If you are travelling to a part of the world in which travellers are advised to take anti-malaria tablets, your GP will prescribe you with a safe one (some are considered unsafe in pregnancy). It's worth taking them, as there is a high risk of miscarriage if you catch malaria.

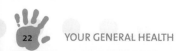

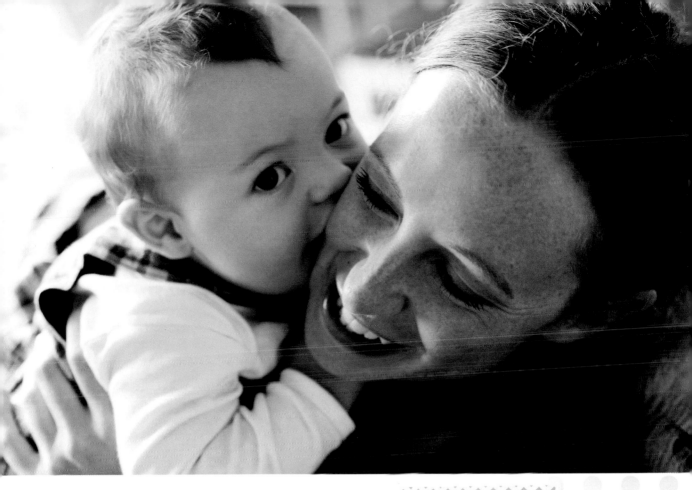

Herbal remedies/complementary treatments

Homeopathy is not clinically trialled as rigorously as medicines, so its safety during pregnancy is uncertain. Herbal remedies should be taken only on the advice of a qualified herbalist who knows you are pregnant, and with the green light from your GP, midwife or obstetrician. Some herbs are dangerous for fetuses. Most herbal teas, however, are safe, and many pregnant women find drinking ginger, chamomile or peppermint tea helpful for alleviating morning sickness.

Reflexology, massage, acupuncture and osteopathy are safe. Many women use them to help them through pregnancy and labour. Ensure your practitioner knows that you are pregnant.

Pre-existing medical conditions

If you have a medical condition, tell your GP or specialist consultant that you are trying for a baby. In the case of a surprise pregnancy, don't stop taking your medication, but let your GP and medical consultant know as soon as possible. They will adjust your medication accordingly. Certain medications are safe during pregnancy, such as topical steroid creams for eczema, inhalers for asthma and statins to lower cholesterol levels. Some drugs are known to have harmful effects. These include steroids in tablet form (dosages may need to change), drugs for high blood pressure such as angiotensin-converting enzyme (ACE) inhibitors, angtiotensin II receptor blockers (ARBs) and thiazide diuretics, diazepam (for anxiety), some antiepilepsy drugs, antiacne drugs (Roaccutane), and certain antidepressants and antipsychotic drugs.

Your trimesters – week by week

Pregnancy is divided into three trimesters, with each one lasting roughly 13 weeks. Your baby develops rapidly throughout pregnancy, and each week brings remarkable changes.

③

1–3

✔ *Start taking a folic acid supplement (ask your GP about daily dosage) to help avoid birth defects in the baby*

✔ *Relax and take gentle exercise in order to support your body*

You won't even know for sure that you are pregnant, yet momentous changes are taking place. A new life has begun and your amazing body is responding rapidly and efficiently to allow it to develop.

What's going on with you?

✦ Did you know that during weeks 1 and 2 of pregnancy you are not actually pregnant? Pregnancy is charted from the first day of the period you had directly before becoming pregnant.

✦ As soon as you become pregnant, your body releases pregnancy hormones (see page 27) to support the new baby's development.

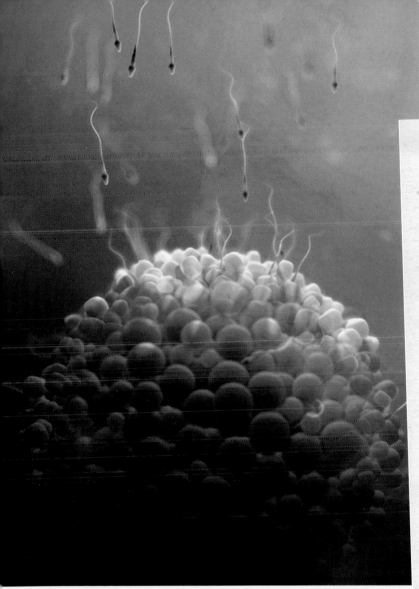

Fertilisation

Each month, two weeks before your period is due, an egg is released from one or both ovaries. For a few days, it moves along the fallopian tube towards the womb, then it disintegrates. If you have sex before it perishes, a sperm may break through its surface to fertilise it, creating a single cell. Fertilisation usually takes place in a fallopian tube. Sperm swim up from the vagina through the cervix, across the womb and into the fallopian tubes.

Multiplying cells

As the single cell continues towards the womb, it splits into two. Each new cell splits into two, and so on, so that the number of cells quickly multiplies. After three to five days, the egg reaches the womb. About a week after fertilisation, it attaches itself to the wall of the womb (a process called 'implantation').

Boy or girl?

Whether your baby is a boy or a girl is determined by the sperm. Both egg and sperm contain half the genes needed to make a human being; when fused, the genes combine to make a full set. The genes that determine a baby's gender are known as 'X' (for a girl) and 'Y' (for a boy) chromosomes. The egg always contains an 'X' chromosome. If the successful sperm also contains an X chromosome, the baby will be a girl. If it contains a Y chromosome, the baby will be a boy.

What's happening to your baby?

✦ During week 3, after fertilisation (see box, right), the new life consists of a bundle of cells. These form into layers. One will become the placenta (which nourishes your baby as he grows), while others will grow into the various parts of his body. One layer becomes the skin, hair, nails, the nervous system and brain. Another becomes the heart, blood vessels, skeleton and bones. The innermost layer will be the digestive and respiratory systems.

✦ Implantation (when the fertilised egg attaches itself to the wall of the womb) takes place towards the end of week 3.

✦ The brain and nervous system have already begun to develop by the end of week 3.

4

✓ Buy a pregnancy test. Good luck!

✓ If you smoke, quit now. Ask your GP for advice or try a local service designed to help pregnant women stop smoking

This week, you can take a pregnancy test, which will now be able to detect the presence of the hormone bhCG (see box, opposite) and determine for sure whether or not you are pregnant.

What's going on with you?

✦ Try not to be anxious while you wait to find out whether you are pregnant. If you have been trying to conceive for a year or more with no luck and you get your period again this month, ask your GP for advice.

✦ A pregnancy test kit, available over the counter from pharmacies, is exactly the same as those used by hospitals and GPs. It will therefore be just as accurate for confirming a pregnancy.

✦ If you are pregnant, hormones are now creating major changes in your body (see opposite). It's unlikely that you will have pregnancy symptoms at this stage; however, you might feel different. Some women say that they have a feeling of calmness or fullness, or simply a feeling of knowing that they are pregnant.

What's happening to your baby?

✦ The embryo (as the baby is known at this stage) is well embedded into the wall of the womb.

✦ A basic blood circulation system is already established.

✦ The embryo could be seen under a powerful microscope as a tiny little bump on the surface of the womb (see picture, opposite). It measures just 2mm across.

"After fertilisation, you might have a little light bleeding, which can happen when the fertilised egg embeds itself into the wall of the womb. Don't be alarmed or confuse it for a period."

Pregnancy hormones

Estrogen helps to thicken the wall of the womb to encourage the embryo to remain embedded. It also stimulates the milk glands in your breasts to grow.

bhCG helps the embryo to remain embedded in the lining of the womb. It speeds up the mother's metabolism, to deliver oxygen around the body more quickly and plentifully. This is necessary because her internal organs grow in size during pregnancy and therefore need more oxygen.

Progesterone helps to regulate the changes in the mother's metabolism. So that her body can deal with the larger quantity of blood flowing through the blood vessels, progesterone creates changes in the circulation system to prevent her blood pressure becoming dangerously high. Progesterone also thickens the 'plug' of mucus that forms in the cervix during early pregnancy, which stops bacteria from entering the womb via the vagina and harming the baby

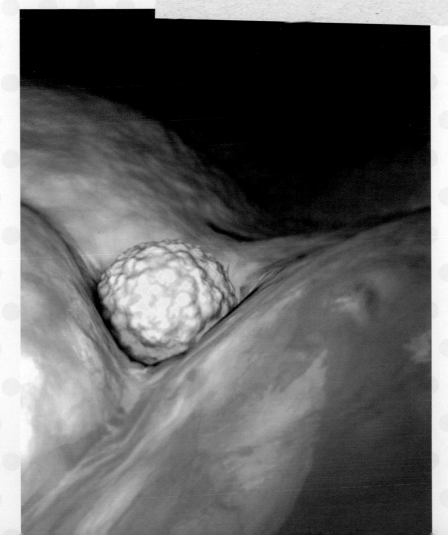

5

✓ Ensure you know which foods to avoid during pregnancy and how to prepare meals hygienically (see pages 12–17)

✓ Buy a vitamin supplement designed for pregnancy, containing folic acid and vitamin D

You may be still coming to terms with being pregnant and the fact that your life is about to change completely. Enormous changes have already taken place inside your body.

What's going on with you?

✦ If you took a pregnancy test last week and it was negative, but you still haven't had your period, try another test this week. It could be that the levels of pregnancy hormones in your bloodstream will now be high enough for the pregnancy test to be able to detect them.

✦ Some jobs bring you into contact with substances (see page 21) or put you in situations that pose a risk to your pregnancy. If your job puts you at risk, your employer is required by law to assess that risk and provide you with a safer job, if necessary, without any loss of pay.

✦ If you are unexpectedly pregnant, don't worry about anything you may have done before you knew you were pregnant that you think might have harmed the baby. Concentrate instead on thinking about how to improve your lifestyle from now on (see pages 12–23) – you can still give your baby a good start in life.

"Don't worry if you've had period-type cramps or an ache in the lower abdomen for the past week, as if you are expecting your period. This is normal. A warm bath may be soothing."

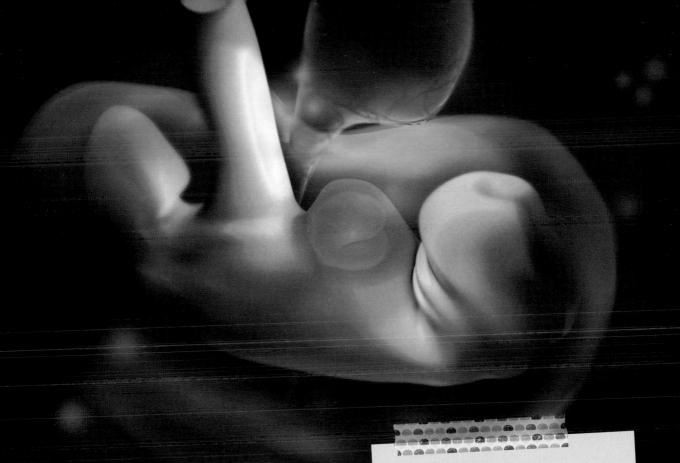

What's happening to your baby?

✦ The baby is now just large enough to be detected by ultrasound scan. She is now covered by a thin layer of skin. Her heart has begun to form. It has a very simple tube-like shape through which blood is already circulating.

✦ The cells that will become the spinal cord are now in place at the back of the body. At one end of the spinal cord is an area consisting of two larger bumps (shown to the right in the picture above) – this is the developing brain.

✦ A very basic digestive system is now in place, running through the centre of the body from top to tail. Eventually, all the digestive organs (such as the stomach and liver) will develop from this tube.

Vitamin D

Approximately 25 per cent of people lack vitamin D, and the percentage is even greater in vegetarians and vegans. You need to be outdoors in natural daylight (not specifically sunshine) for at least 40 minutes per day for your body to produce the amount of vitamin D that it needs in order to take in calcium from the food you eat (which is needed to form your baby's bones). Make sure you spend that much time outdoors every day. Combine it with some gentle exercise and you will have ticked off two good deeds in one hit!

6

✓ If you have had a previous ectopic pregnancy, ask your healthcare provider for a transvaginal scan

✓ If you haven't already done so, reduce your alcohol consumption

✓ Cut down on the number of teas and coffees you drink

Although you are still in the early part of your pregnancy and you may not even know that you are pregnant, your baby's development is marching on at full speed regardless.

What's going on with you?

✦ Extra blood is being pumped to almost every part of your body to help support the pregnancy. The amount of blood directed towards the womb has now doubled because the placenta, the organ that will soon nourish your baby, has begun to grow.

✦ Your vulva, vagina and cervix also receive more blood, which can make them turn a bluish-purple colour. Before pregnancy tests were available, this change in colour was often used by doctors to confirm a new pregnancy.

✦ Your womb has become slightly larger since you conceived and is now roughly the size of a tennis ball. By the end of pregnancy, it will be 20 times heavier than before pregnancy.

What's happening to your baby?

✦ The embryo is now shaped like a comma and resembles a small prawn. It measures 5mm and weighs just 1g.

✦ The cavities that will become the nose and mouth will develop from the bulge at the front section at the top of the embryo. The gill-like folds beneath this bulge will become the face and jaw.

✦ Small, bud-like growths will become limbs.

✦ The heart bulges out from the middle section. It may now be possible to detect a heartbeat by an ultrasound scan.

"Start a pregnancy journal to record your thoughts and feelings throughout pregnancy. You can also keep track of your antenatal appointments and scans, to help you plan ahead."

Early support system

The embryo floats in a protective fluid-filled sac known as the amniotic sac. This grows with the baby and eventually bursts open when your waters break at the end of the pregnancy (see page 104). The placenta has begun to develop and, in the coming weeks, will be ready to nourish your baby until the end of the pregnancy. Until then, the yolk sac provides the necessary blood cells, hormones and nutrients to help the embryo to grow. By the end of this trimester, the yolk sac will have shrivelled and the placenta will have developed enough to take over the job.

The yolk sac and the embryo are enclosed in a membrane known as 'the chorion'. On the outside of the chorion is a bundle of tiny extensions (known as 'chorionic villi') that burrow into the wall of the womb. These will develop into the placenta. They contain blood vessels that allow vital nutrients and gases contained in the mother's blood to pass from the mother to the baby along the umbilical cord, which has begun to develop. The mother's and baby's blood never actually mix, but come close enough in the placenta for this exchange to take place.

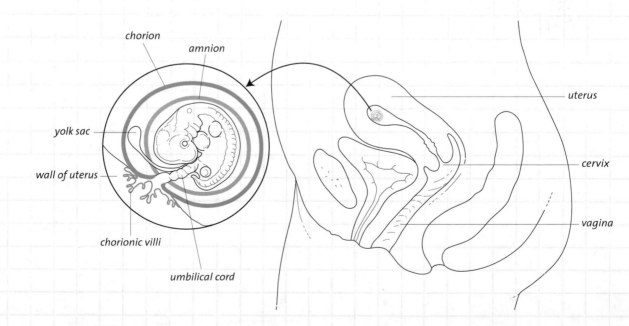

chorion

amnion

yolk sac

wall of uterus

chorionic villi

umbilical cord

uterus

cervix

vagina

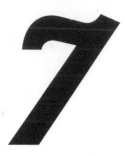

It's time to think about your medical care. There are options available to you within the healthcare system and familiarising yourself with them early on in your pregnancy makes good sense.

> ✓ Fill out and submit the FW8 form (which is available from your GP or midwife) to claim free prescriptions and dental care during pregnancy and the first year after birth

> ✓ Get regular exercise, but listen to your body and don't overdo it

What's going on with you?

✦ Make an appointment to see your GP if you haven't yet done so. Your GP will arrange for you to meet your midwife, who will explain your options for antenatal care and help you to plan your medical care for pregnancy and birth.

✦ You might begin to feel morning sickness around now (see page 35). Women tend to wait until the start of the second trimester to tell people they are pregnant, but it may help to let a few trusted friends and/or a trusted colleague into the secret if you find the morning sickness overwhelming and need support.

What's happening to your baby?

✦ The digestive system is developing and the bowel is taking shape.

✦ Early paddle-shaped hands and feet have now developed.

✦ The embryo's brain is growing rapidly, and the neck and forehead have begun to form. The bones in the face have begun to develop, so the ears, eyes, nose and jaw are more distinct and recognisable.

✦ Your baby's lungs have now begun to develop.

✦ Over the next four weeks, your baby will quadruple in size.

"Start to do your homework on your family's medical and child-bearing histories, so that when you have your booking appointment you have all the information ready."

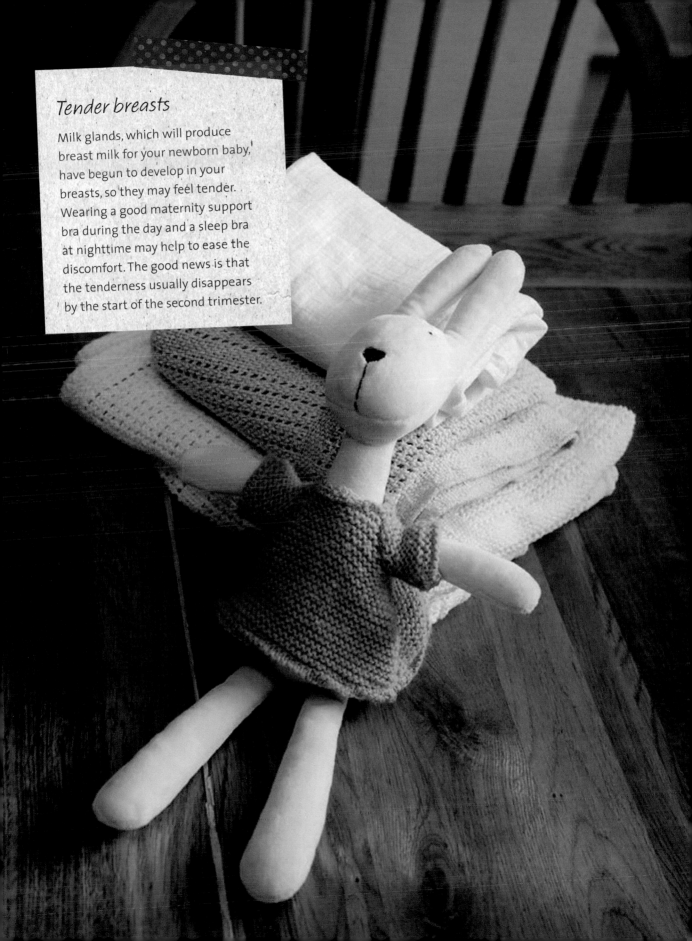

Tender breasts

Milk glands, which will produce breast milk for your newborn baby, have begun to develop in your breasts, so they may feel tender. Wearing a good maternity support bra during the day and a sleep bra at nighttime may help to ease the discomfort. The good news is that the tenderness usually disappears by the start of the second trimester.

8

✔ Take regular rests

✔ Consider a holiday to lift your spirits and allow you to relax

Hormonal changes, combined with anxieties about the future, can make you feel low in the early weeks. Try not to let this get in the way of enjoying your pregnancy.

What's going on with you?

✦ Mood swings (see page 50) are common during early pregnancy. Sometimes you can feel overwhelmed by the major life change that you are going through. Try to remember that many pregnant women experience the same feelings. You are not alone. These feelings will pass soon enough.

✦ By now you may experience pregnancy symptoms such as morning sickness (see opposite), headaches and dizziness (see page 55), tiredness (see page 37), breast tenderness (see page 33) or abdominal aches and pains (see page 85). But don't worry if none of these are present – some women have no symptoms at all.

✦ If you find you are tired at work, build regular rests into your day. Use your lunch break to take a nap if possible, and try to go to bed a little earlier each night.

✦ Don't worry if you find that you are passing urine more often – this is perfectly normal (see page 48).

Food cravings

Many pregnant women develop a longing for certain foods, especially during the first trimester. Salty foods, such as pickled onions, are common cravings, but some women crave unusual substances, such as coal or ice shavings. These cravings are known as 'pica'. It is unlikely that you will crave food that is dangerous to you or your baby, but ask your GP or midwife if you are unsure.

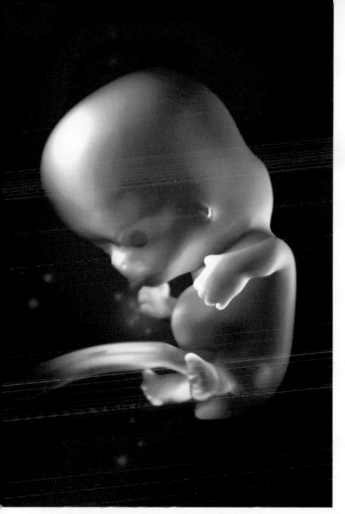

"You'll find your own way to deal with nausea or sickness. Eating little and often helps. If you've gone off fruits and veg, as long as your diet has been healthy, there'll be nutrient stores to nourish the baby."

What's happening to your baby?

✦ Your baby now measures 16mm.

✦ The arms and shoulders have taken shape. The elbows can bend and the wrists can be identified. Fingers have begun to form. The legs are less developed than the arms.

✦ There are now ten tooth buds in the jaw that will develop into milk teeth in the future.

Morning sickness

Most pregnant women experience morning sickness, which can happen at any time of day, despite the name. Symptoms range from mild nausea to frequent and severe vomiting. If you have been pregnant before, you might find your symptoms are different this time. Severe vomiting, while distressing, does not harm the baby; if you cannot keep fluids down for 24 hours, contact your midwife or GP to ensure that you don't become dehydrated. If you are really suffering, you'll be pleased to know that in many cases, symptoms ease between weeks 12 and 15. The following tips may help you find some relief:

✦ eat little and often – a small meal every hour or two may be easier to digest
✦ stick to plain, starchy foods, such as crackers, oatcakes, toast and plain pasta
✦ keep a plain, starchy snack by your bed, to give you a boost when you wake up
✦ if you have gone off many foods, fill up on breakfast cereals that are fortified with calcium and vitamins, with skimmed milk
✦ avoid acidic fruit juices, fatty, rich or spicy foods, and cooking smells
✦ wear an acupressure wristband (available from pharmacies)
✦ take as much rest as possible.

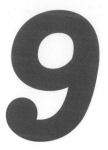

9

✓ Get professionally fitted for a maternity bra

✓ Begin considering your birth options (see pages 10–11)

Although you won't be able to feel it, your baby may well have started making tiny movements. His rapid development puts a great strain on your body, and you may be feeling exhausted.

What's going on with you?

✦ Hormonal changes will have made your breasts larger, and they may feel tender and heavy. Buy a few maternity bras to give your breasts proper support. You can use these until towards the end of your pregnancy, when your breasts will increase in size again, in order to produce milk.

✦ Your nipples and the circles of skin around them (the areolae) are darker, with perhaps a lighter circle of colouring around each areola. The areolae themselves are larger. Tiny bumps may be visible around the nipples that might leak a clear fluid as the milk ducts prepare for breastfeeding. The veins on your breasts may be more visible.

What's happening to your baby?

✦ The embryo measures 23mm from crown (the top of the head) to rump (the baby's bottom). The body is slowly straightening out and lengthening.

✦ The brain is now four times larger than it was three weeks ago. The nervous system is developing – nerve cells are multiplying, and special cells that join the nerve cells (allowing messages to pass between body and brain) are forming.

✦ Your baby's unique facial features are forming. The eyelids have begun to develop, and the tip of the nose has taken shape.

✦ The heart now has the basic structure of a human heart, with four chambers. Blood flows through it and is pumped around the body. The heart beats at 160 beats per minute – twice the speed of an adult heart.

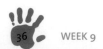

"It is said in some cultures that baby girls steal your beauty! If your skin is suffering due to hormone changes, drink plenty of water and invest in a lovely new foundation as you revisit this concern from your teens."

Tiredness

Pregnancy puts your body under a lot of strain, which will leave you feeling exhausted at times. Don't be alarmed if you feel wiped out at the end of the day – this is entirely normal, especially during the first trimester. Take a nap in the middle of the day, go to bed earlier and reduce your normal activities and social life to alleviate the tiredness. Some women, particularly those who are usually very active and busy, can find the tiredness highly frustrating. Try to remember that this is a temporary state. Your body is working hard to support your baby's development and needs appropriate rest.

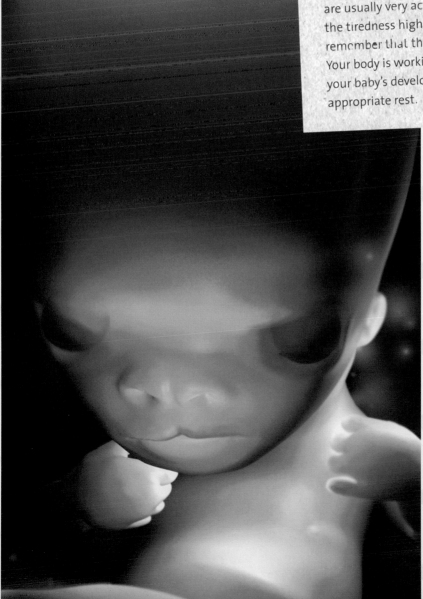

10

✓ Drink plenty of water and eat melons and cucumbers to stay well hydrated

✓ If you haven't done so already, establish an appropriate exercise routine

✓ If you are constipated, eat plenty of fibre (found in wholegrain foods and fresh fruits and vegetables)

"Read up on screening tests so that you can let your midwife know whether you would like to have any."

This week (the last week in which your baby is described as an embryo) marks the end of a major stage of development, after which the baby is much less vulnerable.

What's going on with you?
✦ Even though you can't yet detect the increase in size, your womb is now roughly 10cm in diameter. It has grown from the size of your fist to the size of a grapefruit.

✦ Many women experience heavier vaginal discharge during pregnancy. It should be odourless, clear or milky, with a mucus-like consistency. Contact your GP or midwife if it smells, becomes yellow or feels itchy, which may indicate thrush.

✦ Your body needs to take in 40 per cent more air, which is directed towards the baby, womb and placenta, so you might be feeling breathless. If, however, you experience any pain upon breathing in, speak to your GP or midwife.

What's happening to your baby?
✦ The baby now measures 32mm from crown to rump and weighs 3–5g.

✦ All the major organs will have taken shape by the end of this week.

✦ The hands have fingers with touch pads at the ends. The legs have knees, and the feet are developing toes.

✦ The head is well formed, with nostrils and an upper lip. A tongue has taken shape, and taste buds have begun to form. The outer ear progresses, and the inner ear (which allows for hearing and balance) is fully formed.

✦ The digestive system is developing rapidly. The bowel is developed enough in length to become looped and coiled.

✦ Muscle development allows the baby to make movements that are a little more graceful than the previous jerky attempts.

The booking appointment

The first appointment of your antenatal care should take place during weeks 10–12. The midwife will note your personal and family medical history and establish your estimated delivery date (EDD) from the date of your last period. Your BMI (body mass index) will be measured using your weight and height. The information is noted in a book referred to as 'hand-held notes', which you keep with you and take to all your antenatal appointments. You will be asked some personal questions, for example, about previous terminations or drug use. If you feel uncomfortable answering these questions, remember that providing accurate information better allows the midwife to assess any risks to your pregnancy. Simply ask her not to write down any sensitive information in your notes. She will check your blood pressure and arrange for you to have a blood test to establish your blood group, your rhesus factor and rubella immunity, and screen for HIV, hepatitis, syphilis and anaemia, which could all affect the baby. The midwife will also test your urine for any signs of infection.

11

✓ *Start researching local hospitals and birth centres*

Your baby is now classed as a fetus. Her body and organs, which until now have been taking shape, will grow rapidly over the coming weeks.

What's going on with you?

✦ If you've been suffering from morning sickness and tiredness, you might find your symptoms easing at this point.

✦ This is a good time to begin to think about the type of birth you want. Do you prefer to give birth in a hospital or is a home birth for you? How do you feel about pain relief? Who would you like as your birth partner? Over the next few weeks you can make decisions for your birth, then write your birth plan (see pages 100–101) into your hand-held notes.

✦ You and your partner may feel anxious about coping financially once the baby is born. Discuss your worries with one another, and ask other parents about their strategies so that you can plan for life after birth.

What's happening to your baby?

✦ The baby now measures 42mm from crown to rump, and her shape is recognisably human.

✦ Her head is still proportionally larger than the rest of her body, but its growth will now slow down, to allow the rest of the body to catch up. Her neck lengthens, and her jawline is clearly visible.

✦ Her bones are made up of soft bone tissue (cartilage) that is hardening – this process will continue throughout pregnancy and into her childhood and adolescence.

✦ The internal sex organs (ovaries in girls, testes in boys) are developed, but the external sex organs (the clitoris or penis) are still developing, and you cannot yet tell whether the baby is a boy or a girl.

The placenta

For the past few weeks, your body has been growing an amazing organ especially to support your baby's development. This organ is now functioning well (although it continues to grow throughout pregnancy) and, by week 13, will be solely responsible for supplying your baby with air and nourishment, and passing out her body's waste products. The placenta is attached to the wall of the womb and is connected to the baby via the umbilical cord. The baby's blood vessels pass through the umbilical cord into the placenta and approach the mother's blood vessels, but the mother's and baby's blood vessels are separated by the intervillous space (see diagram, below). The mother's blood leaks into this space and pools around the baby's blood vessels. The baby's blood vessels extract oxygen, nutrients and fluids from these pools of maternal blood and pass back carbon dioxide and other waste products from the baby. These in turn enter the maternal blood vessels and are expelled from the mother's body along with its own waste products.

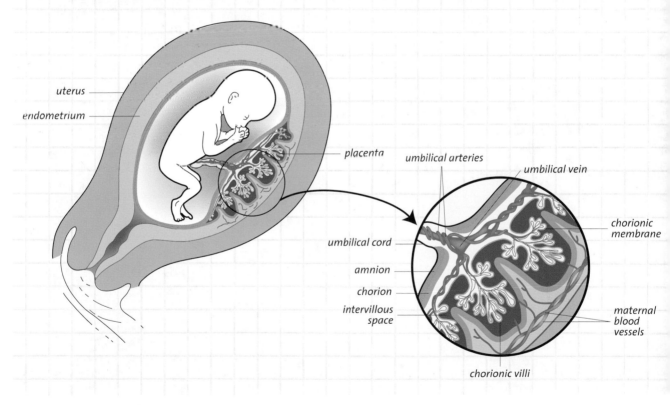

uterus
endometrium
placenta
umbilical arteries
umbilical vein
chorionic membrane
umbilical cord
amnion
chorion
intervillous space
maternal blood vessels
chorionic villi

"Now that the nausea is subsiding, try not to eat for two! Digestion is slower than normal, allowing more nutrients to be absorbed, so choose the most nutritious foods."

12

✓ Join a pregnancy exercise class in your local area

✓ Buy a good maternity sports bra and supportive footwear for exercising safely

You'll may well have your first ultrasound scan this week and will finally 'see' your baby. This is an exciting moment! You and your partner may begin to bond with your unborn baby now you've seen he is really there.

What's going on with you?

✦ Once you've had your first ultrasound scan (see box, opposite), your pregnancy can seem more of a reality and you may feel very excited! Now might be the right time to share your news with others; statistically speaking, you are unlikely to lose the baby at this stage. If you purchased a scan picture, you have a 'photo' to share along with the good news!

✦ With the easing of morning sickness and rise of energy levels, this is the perfect time to start a regular exercise regime, to help your body cope with the demands of pregnancy, prepare you for the physical challenge of giving birth and lift your spirits. Whichever type of exercise you opt for, ensure that it is appropriate for pregnancy (see page 18).

What's happening to your baby?

✦ Your baby measures 54mm from crown to rump and weighs 14g.

✦ His hands and feet are no longer webbed and his clearly defined fingers have tiny fingernails.

✦ In your baby's jaw, 32 tooth buds for his permanent teeth are beginning to form.

✦ His eyelids can now meet, and his eyes begin to take on colour.

✦ The thin, see-through skin now has a fine covering of hair.

✦ Your baby responds to touch with reflex reactions. For instance, he may move in response to something being pressed on your tummy.

✦ His digestive system continues to develop – the mouth, stomach and intestines are now linked. The kidneys (which produce urine) are mature enough to allow him to take in amniotic fluid and pass it out as urine.

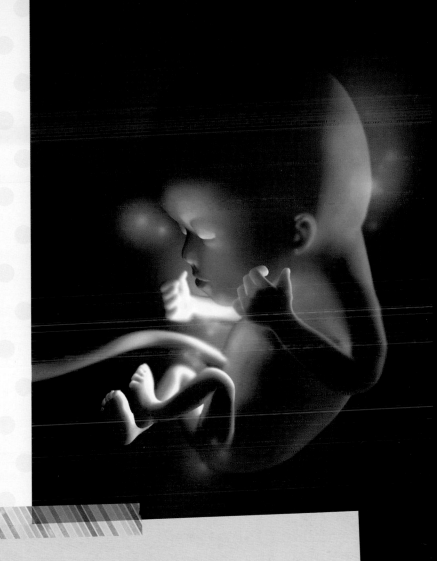

"Take change for the car park with you to your scan, along with a loved one to share the moment with. Don't be late – scans are rarely rearranged, so you'll have missed your opportunity for the most accurate first trimester screening."

The dating scan

Your first ultrasound scan in pregnancy is known as the 'dating scan' because it helps to establish the exact gestational age of your baby (i.e., exactly how long it has been since fertilisation). Fetuses develop at the same rate, so the scan allows the sonographer (the person performing the scan) to see how far along you are in your pregnancy. This is useful if you are unsure of when the first day of your last period was, or if your periods were irregular. Two measurements are taken: the crown–rump length (CRL) and the biparietal diameter (BPD) – the measurement across the parietal bones on each side of the head. These are used to calculate your estimated delivery date (EDD). The sonographer also measures the heart rate and checks the position of the placenta. You will see your baby's heartbeat, limbs, head and spine. You'll be asked to drink lots of water before the scan, as a full bladder pushes the uterus into a position that produces a clear image. The sonographer applies special gel to your tummy, then holds a hand-held device against the device and moves it gently across the area. The technology uses sound waves to produce a picture of the baby on a screen. The process is painless and completely safe. You will be given the option of buying a scan image to take home with you.

13

✓ Start writing a list of all the things you will need to have ready for your baby

✓ Plan your meals and snacks for a healthy, balanced diet

This is the last week of the first trimester, and you are about to embark on the part of your pregnancy in which you'll have the most energy and vitality. If this is your first pregnancy, you may be starting to show.

What's going on with you?

✦ Your womb is roughly 12cm wide, and the top of it is now high up enough in your abdomen to reach above the pelvic bone. Your midwife can now feel it when touching your tummy.

✦ As morning sickness diminishes, your appetite returns with a vengeance! Be careful not to overeat, as you can easily put on too much weight. Ideally, you should increase by no more than 1kg in the first trimester, 6kg in the second trimester and 6kg in the third trimester. You should be eating between 2,000 and 2,500 calories per day.

✦ Your breasts will have become much larger over the past few weeks. The growth now slows down until the end of pregnancy. Your nipples may have become larger and more erect.

What's happening to your baby?

✦ The facial features continue to develop – the ears have migrated further up the sides of the head, and the eyes have moved further towards the front of the face.

✦ The body is straightening out slowly.

✦ Your baby's taste buds have developed further.

✦ The brain is developing at quite a pace, as are the muscles, allowing your baby to make a greater range of movements.

✦ Your baby makes reflex facial movements, which give her expressions such as grinning or frowning.

Nuchal translucency scan

This scan allows your healthcare providers to establish how high the chances are of your baby having Down's syndrome. It cannot tell you for certain if your baby does have Down's, but if the test result indicates that your baby has a high chance of having Down's syndrome, you can go on to have further testing to find out for sure (see page 137). The scan must be done between weeks 11 and 14 of your pregnancy. It measures the thickness of the fold of skin at the back of the baby's neck. If the thickness is 3mm or more, there is a higher chance that the baby has Down's syndrome. A baby without Down's might still have a high measurement, and a baby with a lower measurement might still have Down's syndrome. The measurement and your age, combined with the results of the serum test, if you have it (see page 137), will be used to calculate the overall risk factor.

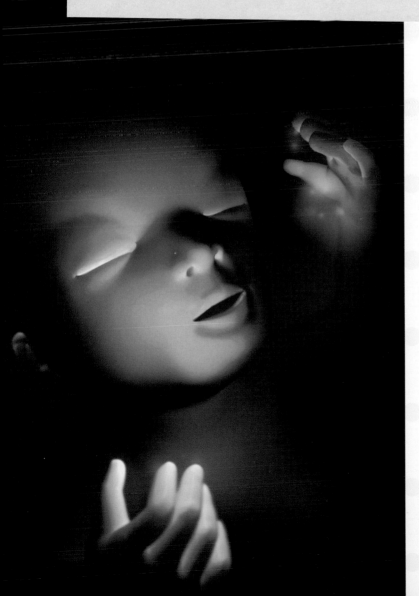

"As your baby's taste buds develop, they are tuning in to the foods that you are eating, which can influence her likes and dislikes during weaning. This is a good time to practise what you'll soon be preaching, and eat your greens!"

14

> ✓ *Arrange to have the screening blood test for Down's syndrome (see page 136–7)*

You are now at the start of the second trimester, during which the fetus will develop into a fully formed baby. As he becomes bigger and stronger, so will his movements and, soon, you will start to feel them.

What's going on with you?

✦ For most women, the second trimester is the most enjoyable part of pregnancy. Tiredness and morning sickness are in the past, and the risk of miscarriage is greatly reduced. Your bump becomes visible, but it won't become large enough in this trimester to stop you from doing what you want to do. Resolve to enjoy this golden period!

✦ Many women have an increased sex drive in pregnancy, particularly in the second trimester. Sex is perfectly safe during pregnancy (see page 63), but as your bump becomes larger you'll need to find sexual positions that will allow for its size.

What's happening to your baby?

✦ The baby now measures 80mm from crown to rump and weighs 45g.

✦ The genitals have developed enough to tell the sex by ultrasound scan.

✦ The fully developed legs are growing quickly, as are the arms, which are long enough for the hands to be able to meet.

✦ Your baby's body can now produce its own red blood cells (up until now, it has been receiving them from the placenta).

✦ His heartbeat has slowed down and currently beats at 110–160 beats per minute, which is still faster than the average adult's heartbeat (70 bpm). It will continue to decrease during pregnancy and childhood, and will reach the adult rate by the time your child is roughly ten years old.

✦ Although his eyelids are still shut, his eyes are now sensitive to light.

✦ During much of pregnancy, your baby's body will be covered in fine, downy hair (see page 62). This begins to develop now and is already present on the eyebrows and upper lip.

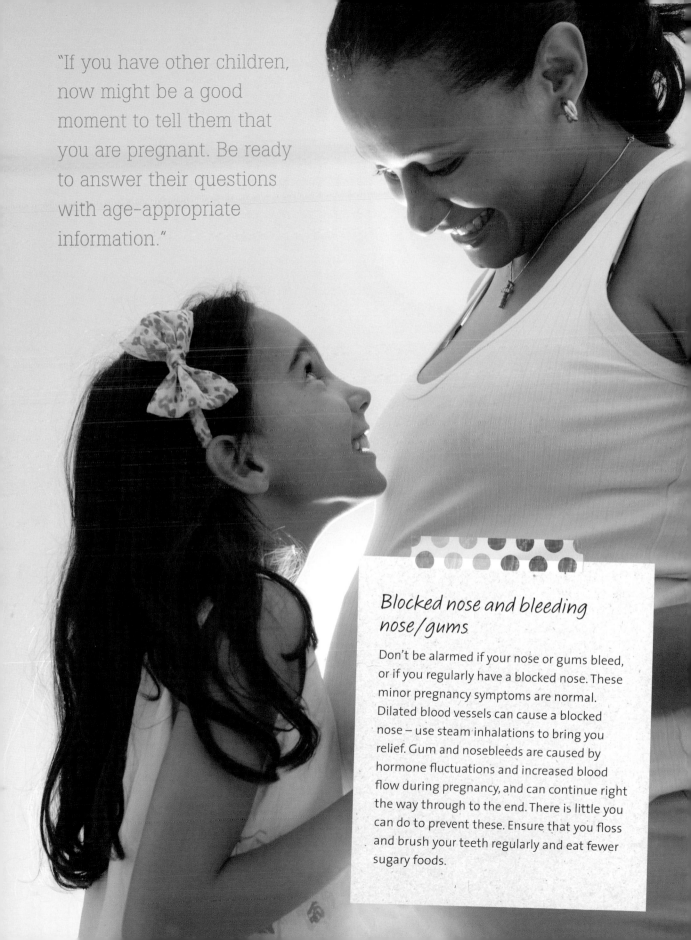

"If you have other children, now might be a good moment to tell them that you are pregnant. Be ready to answer their questions with age-appropriate information."

Blocked nose and bleeding nose/gums

Don't be alarmed if your nose or gums bleed, or if you regularly have a blocked nose. These minor pregnancy symptoms are normal. Dilated blood vessels can cause a blocked nose – use steam inhalations to bring you relief. Gum and nosebleeds are caused by hormone fluctuations and increased blood flow during pregnancy, and can continue right the way through to the end. There is little you can do to prevent these. Ensure that you floss and brush your teeth regularly and eat fewer sugary foods.

15

✓ *Sign up to antenatal (parent craft) classes*

From now until week 18, your baby is in a phase of rapid growth. Meanwhile, you are likely to be blooming – you're looking and feeling your best. Enjoy the compliments!

What's going on with you?

✦ Over the coming weeks, your circulation system undergoes enormous changes. You will have significantly more blood pumping through your heart. The heart itself increases slightly in size and pumps with more power, in order to move this greater blood supply around your body. At this point in pregnancy, about a quarter of your blood flow is sent to the womb to support the baby's growth. Due to hormonal changes, your blood pressure may actually be lower than it was before pregnancy.

✦ You may by now be enjoying some of the beneficial side effects of pregnancy. Receiving a boosted blood supply gives the skin a healthy glow (often referred to as 'pregnancy glow'). Also, the hair tends to look more glossy, and it becomes thicker because less of it falls out on a daily basis than usual, due to hormonal changes. (On the down side, you'll shed more hair after pregnancy to make up for what you would have lost during those months.) The nails become healthier and stronger, too.

Frequent urination

You may feel the urge to pee more often than you did before pregnancy. At the beginning, this is due to a change in the blood supply to your kidneys. Later on in pregnancy, it might be because your growing womb is pressing down on the bladder, which gives you the feeling of needing to pee (although you may pass very little urine each time you go). If you find it inconvenient to be making frequent trips to the toilet, try reducing your intake of coffee, tea and colas, as they cause the body to produce more urine than other drinks. Drink water and herbal teas instead.

What's happening to your baby?

✦ This week, your baby will make the first basic movements that mimic breathing. These will continue over the next few weeks, which allows the baby to develop the muscles around her chest needed for breathing and to expand the lungs.

✦ Your baby's spine is now fully formed.

✦ Her movements are becoming more coordinated as her muscles continue to develop, enabling her to perform some sophisticated actions (although these are still reflex actions, rather than deliberate ones). For example, she may suck her thumb if it accidentally touches her mouth.

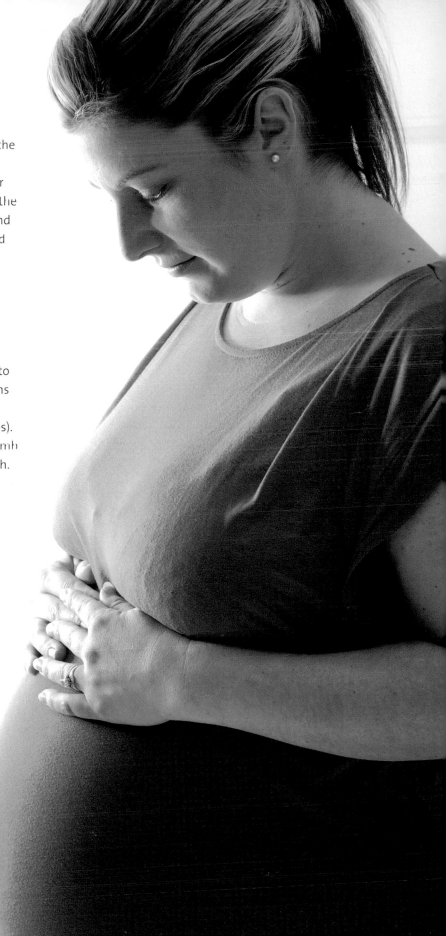

16

✓ Start your birth plan (see page 100-101)

✓ Practise pelvic-floor exercises (see page 19). If you haven't already, get into a habit of regular practice

Antenatal appointments take place roughly once a month at this stage of pregnancy, so it may now be time to see your midwife again, to check on the baby's progress.

What's going on with you?

✦ It's likely that your second antenatal appointment takes place this week. You'll have the usual blood and urine tests, and a chance to hear your baby's heartbeat. If you have any concerns or questions, raise them with your midwife. You may have been thinking about your birth plan for a while now (see page 100-101). Your midwife can provide you with information and guide you on which choices are right for you.

✦ Your midwife may mention that your urine contains small amounts of sugar and protein. This is nothing to be alarmed about. It happens because the kidneys are working harder than normal – by the end of pregnancy, they are filtering 60 per cent more blood than they were before pregnancy.

Mood swings

You could find your emotions shifting dramatically from one moment to the next and that you suddenly feel angry, tearful and grumpy. Don't worry – this is perfectly normal during pregnancy and is caused by hormonal changes. Talk to friends and family about your feelings, and get support when you are feeling blue. Try to remember that these feelings will pass. Do your best not to lose your temper with your partner. Let him know that your feelings are temporary and normal in pregnancy, so that he can support you. Remember that he must have his own feelings of anxiety about supporting you through the rest of the pregnancy and the birth and fulfilling his role as a parent, especially if this is his first child. Make a point of talking openly with one another so that you remain close.

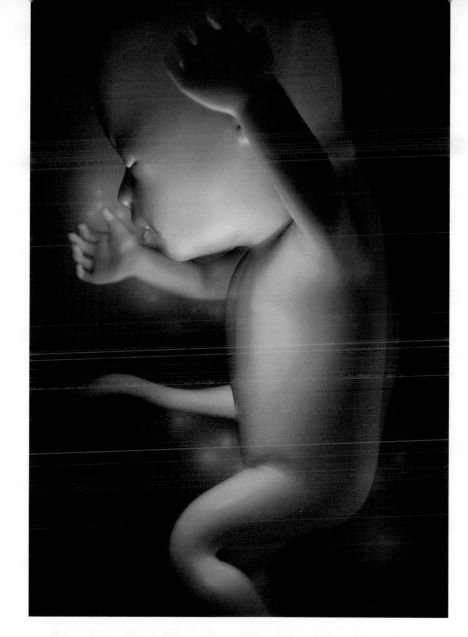

"It's a good idea to write down any questions you have for your midwife, so you don't forget to ask them at your appointment. And don't forget your urine sample."

What's happening to your baby?

✦ Your baby measures 12cm from crown to rump and weighs 110g. Although his body has no fat on it and you can see his blood vessels and some bones through his skin, he now looks decidedly like a baby.

✦ He can now make slow eye movements.

✦ Tiny toenails begin to appear on his toes.

✦ With boy fetuses, the penis and scrotum are fully formed and clearly visible. With girl fetuses, the vagina and fallopian tubes begin to form at this point.

17

✓ If you are in a high-risk group for high blood pressure, you can reduce the risk by taking regular exercise

By now it will be difficult to hide the fact that you are pregnant. If you haven't yet told people, it's likely that they will guess very soon, no matter how baggy your clothes may be!

What's going on with you?

✦ Pregnant women tend to share the news of their pregnancy towards the start of the second trimester, once the chances of miscarriage are greatly reduced. It's wonderful to share your joy with others, but be prepared for some people wanting to share with you in return their advice about pregnancy and childbirth. Also prepare yourself for the fact that some people will now see you differently. A childless friend might feel sad at the idea of losing you as a partner in fun, or an employer might have a less-than-ideal response to losing a valued member of staff to maternity leave. Try to respond with sensitivity, but don't allow other people's negative reactions to hurt your feelings.

✦ If you are over 40, overweight, diabetic or a smoker, you are at greater risk of developing high blood pressure or pre-eclampsia, both of which are dangerous to the baby if left unmanaged. Your midwife will check your blood pressure at each antenatal appointment and will advise you on signs and symptoms to look out for.

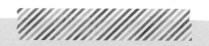

Sweats and hot flushes

Due to hormonal changes and also changes in your circulation, you are likely to feel hotter during pregnancy than you did before. This can be particularly challenging if you are pregnant over the summer months. Wear loose layers that you can shed to allow you to cool down quickly, and stick to natural fibres such as cotton or linen, which don't cause sweating as much as synthetic fibres. Open windows to keep a draught flowing through the room. If you suffer from frequent hot flushes, try regular exercise to improve your circulation.

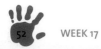

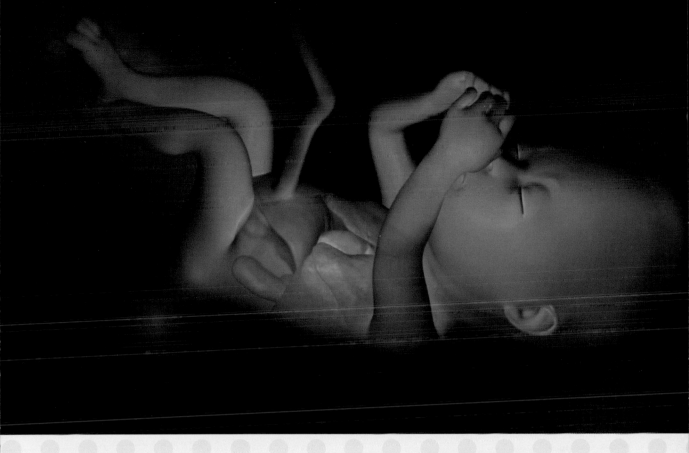

What's happening to your baby?

✦ Your baby's lungs and digestive system are now fully developed and have begun to mature.

✦ The nervous system has matured further, and messages between the brain and the rest of the body now travel with more speed, allowing for increasingly sophisticated movements. The baby moves around inside the amniotic sac due to her increasing physical abilities. She is still quite small, which means that there is plenty of space for her movements.

✦ Her eyes are now closer to the front of her face.

✦ The baby's head is still proportionally very large, but the rest of the body is slowly catching up. At this point in the pregnancy, the head accounts for just under one-third of the body length.

"Watch out for light fluttering sensations, which indicate your baby is moving. These short episodes may be felt only every couple of days at this stage, but you will in time come to recognise your baby's pattern of movement and to what she responds."

18

> ✓ *Research baby carriers and slings, and select those that seem right for you and your partner*

The baby's movements (known as 'quickening') are usually felt at around this time, although first-time mothers may not become aware of the sensations until around week 20. The movements may feel like a fluttering feeling deep in your belly, which is easily mistaken for wind!

What's going on with you?

✦ Your breasts are preparing for breastfeeding, and milk ducts are developing. The areolae (the darker circles of skin directly around the nipples) have increased in size and may leak a clear, yellowish liquid, especially if you've had a baby before.

✦ Your womb has expanded so much that the top of it (known as the 'fundus') is now halfway between your pubic bone and your navel.

✦ You may suffer side effects caused by the increased blood flow during pregnancy, such as feeling hot and sweaty (see page 52), stuffy nose (see page 47), varicose veins (see page 93), haemorrhoids (see page 91), nosebleeds and gum bleeds (see page 47). While some symptoms are dramatic, they are usually harmless, so don't be alarmed. There are often measures you can take to make yourself more comfortable.

What's happening to your baby?

✦ Your baby measures 14cm from crown to rump and weighs 200g.

✦ His ears have developed enough for him to be able to hear. This is a good time for you and your partner to start talking to him so that he will recognise you voice when he is born.

✦ Your baby's bones continue to harden throughout the body. In his head, the bones of the face are now formed, and the nose has developed further. The ears have moved into their final positions.

✦ In female fetuses, the ovaries are now developed.

✦ Your baby's range of movements is increasing (see picture, opposite).

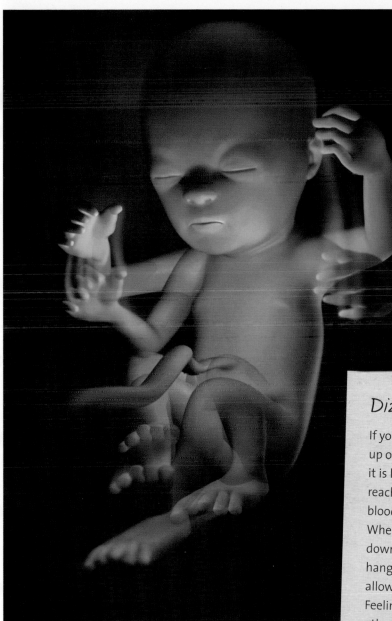

Dizziness

If you become dizzy while standing up or when standing up suddenly, it is likely there is too little blood reaching your brain, as much of your blood supply is directed to the womb. Whenever you feel dizzy, try lying down, or sitting down with your head hanging between your legs, which allows the blood to flow to the head. Feeling dizzy while sitting, on the other hand, may indicate low blood sugar levels, so have a drink and snack.

"Explore exercise classes for pregnant women. Try yoga, Pilates and aquanatal groups to strengthen your core muscles. It will also bring you into contact with other mums."

19

✓ Consider a holiday while it's still easy and safe to travel

✓ Attend the fetal anomaly scan (weeks 18–20)

This is the perfect time to consider a holiday, while it is relatively easy to travel, airlines still allow you to board a flight and you are not too big to make the most of your break.

What's going on with you?

✦ Being pregnant has its highs and lows. During the highs, you feel full of excitement about the future, but during the lows it's easy to feel anxious about how you will cope with motherhood. Talking to others will help you to gain some perspective on your challenges. Taking a holiday might be the perfect way to relieve anxieties and allows you a final fling with freedom before the baby comes. Take your hand-held notes with you, and familiarise yourself with the location of the local maternity unit at your destination, in case of emergency.

✦ You may have felt a few twinges of pain in the tummy area during the first trimester as the ligaments in your pelvis that hold the womb in place adapted to the increasing weight and size by stretching. These aches and pains may well continue into the second trimester, particularly in the pelvis and lower back. However, if the pain comes on suddenly or is severe, appears only on one side, or is constant or feels like cramp, contact your GP immediately.

What's happening to your baby?

✦ The growth spurt that took place from around week 15 now eases and, from now until around week 22, growth will be slow.

✦ Around this week, the fetus's legs arrive at the length they will be when she is born.

✦ Your baby's skin is now releasing a thick, white waxy substance called 'vernix caseosa'. This coats the skin so that it doesn't become waterlogged with amniotic fluid. The coating also protects the skin from damage caused by scratches from your baby's fingernails.

✦ Fat has now started to build up under the baby's skin.

Fetal anomaly scan

Performed during weeks 18–20, your second ultrasound scan will take roughly 20 minutes. This time, you won't need a full bladder because there is enough amniotic fluid in the womb to produce a good 'picture'. This scan is done to check that all is well with the baby and that she is growing at the proper rate. To do this, the sonographer takes a variety of measurements and compares these to average measurements. They also check specific physical features such as the heart, internal organs, brain, skull and spine, limbs and face, to ensure that there are no defects such as a cleft lip, spina bifida or major kidney or heart problems. The sonographer also checks the position of the placenta. If they cannot see everything they need to check, you may be asked to walk around a little to give the baby a chance to shift into a better position. Abnormalities can't be detected for certain by this scan, but if the results indicate a problem your antenatal care team will provide support and guidance. The sonographer may be able to see whether the baby is a boy or a girl, but some hospitals have a policy not to share this information with parents, so you might not be told, even if you want to know! If it's important to you to find out, you can pay to get a scan done privately.

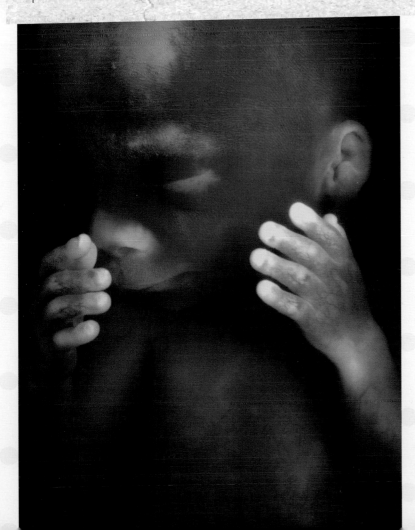

"Try not to worry about abnormalities – the risk itself is very low in healthy women, and in many cases abnormalities can be surgically corrected."

20

> ✔ Buy maternity clothes

> ✔ Start to plan your baby's bedroom, and research the type of cot you want for him

Congratulations – you are halfway through your pregnancy! More than likely, your bump will now be obvious. If you haven't already done so, it's time to invest in some maternity clothes.

What's going on with you?

✦ Your heart is now pumping roughly 7 litres of blood around the body per minute (it pumped 4 litres per minute prior to pregnancy).

✦ Some women develop temporary yet painful conditions such as carpal tunnel syndrome (see page 64) at this stage of pregnancy. In most cases, these conditions recede over time once the baby is born.

✦ You may have already felt your baby moving around, but, if you haven't, you will at around this time. Watch out for fluttery sensations that feel like butterflies in your stomach.

What's happening to your baby?

✦ Your baby measures 16cm from crown to rump and weighs 320g.

✦ His nervous system is developing in leaps and bounds, and his movements have become more sophisticated and precise. He may now be making deliberate movements, rather than only reflex actions. For instance, if something presses against your abdomen, he might respond by moving away from the place where he feels the pressure on the inside.

✦ His bones continue to develop, as do the internal organs. The baby's immune system is functioning well.

✦ Although his eyelids are still closed, his eyeballs can move from side to side, and his eyes are becoming progressively more sensitive to light.

✦ Your baby can move his tongue in and out of his mouth. His taste buds are now capable of distinguishing sweet and bitter flavours.

✦ In baby girls, the uterus is fully developed, and the vagina is taking shape. The ovaries already contain six to seven million eggs.

"Look into booking antenatal classes now. Dads-to-be find them helpful for preparing them for the end of pregnancy, labour, delivery and bringing a new baby home."

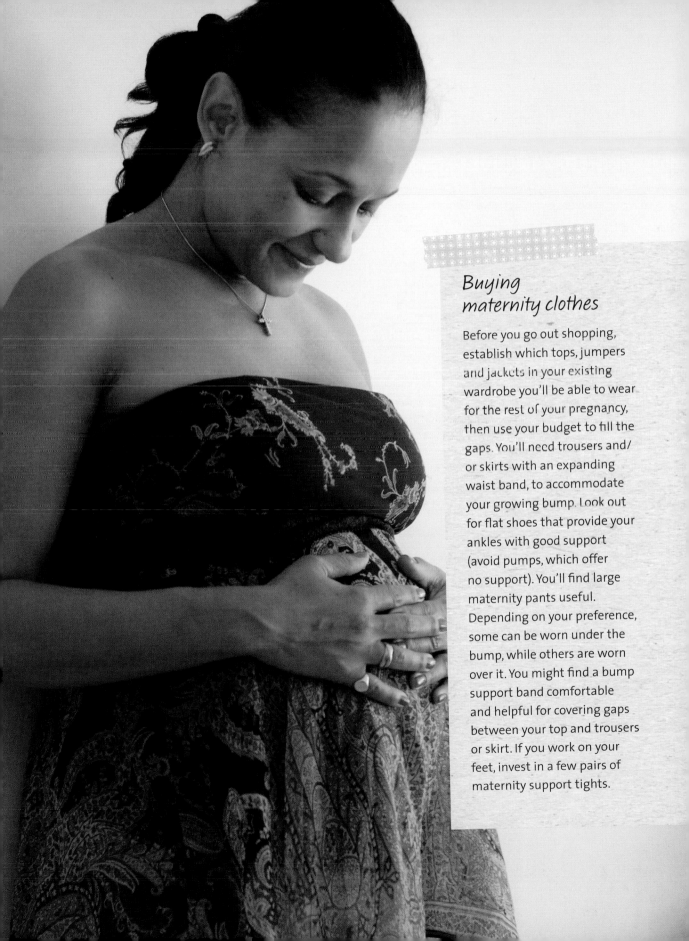

Buying maternity clothes

Before you go out shopping, establish which tops, jumpers and jackets in your existing wardrobe you'll be able to wear for the rest of your pregnancy, then use your budget to fill the gaps. You'll need trousers and/ or skirts with an expanding waist band, to accommodate your growing bump. Look out for flat shoes that provide your ankles with good support (avoid pumps, which offer no support). You'll find large maternity pants useful. Depending on your preference, some can be worn under the bump, while others are worn over it. You might find a bump support band comfortable and helpful for covering gaps between your top and trousers or skirt. If you work on your feet, invest in a few pairs of maternity support tights.

21

✓ Put a note in your diary to pick up a MAT B1 certificate when you are 24 weeks so you can claim Statutory Maternity Pay

This is a good time to consider when to tell your employer that you are pregnant. You can also start to think about when to begin your maternity leave and how to tackle the subject with your boss.

What's going on with you?

✦ Familiarise yourself with your maternity rights and benefits. The Department for Work and Pensions (DWP) has the most up-to-date information about maternity benefits (including maternity pay) on its website (www.gov.uk). The Citizens Advice Bureau has a good leaflet about maternity rights and benefits on its website (www.adviceguide.org.uk). Your own company may offer more than the statutory requirements, so check your contract. Now is the time to decide when to tell your employer that you are pregnant and think about your maternity leave options (see box, opposite).

✦ The top of the womb (the fundus) is at the level of your navel.

✦ You might find your skin feels dry and itchy. Don't worry – this is a normal part of pregnancy and is caused by hormonal changes. Moisturise affected skin regularly.

✦ The size of your growing bump may force you to change the type of exercise you have been doing up until now. Avoid abdominal exercises, and if you enjoy resistance training ensure that the weights you use are light (see page 18). It's safe to continue with aerobic exercises such as swimming, cycling and brisk walking. If you like yoga, pilates, or exercise classes at the gym, ensure that the instructor knows you are pregnant.

"Invest in a moisturiser that is safe in pregnancy, and start a regime to help your skin cope with the growth of your abdomen and reduce stretch marks. Enjoy the me-time it gives you."

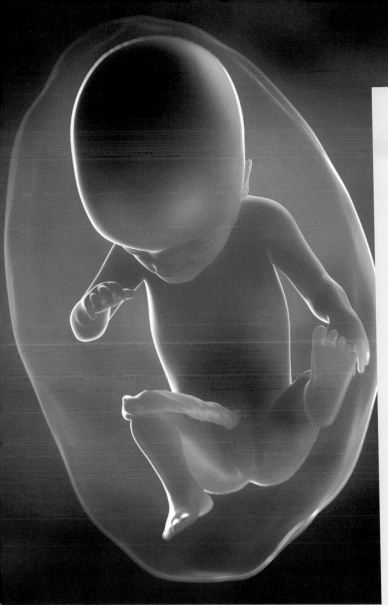

Considering maternity leave

By law, you do not have to tell your employer that you are pregnant until 15 weeks before your due date (i.e. in week 25), at the latest. So your first consideration will be when to tell your boss that you are pregnant. Think about when you will want to begin and end your maternity leave. (Legally, you are entitled to maternity leave of 52 weeks, although not all of this will be paid leave.) There will be a number of factors that will influence your decision, such as:

✦ how your health is, how your pregnancy is progressing and any advice your midwife or GP has given you concerning your health and pregnancy
✦ your financial situation
✦ your professional standing and position within your company
✦ your partner's work situation
✦ whether you have other children
✦ which childcare options are available to you
✦ whether you intend to return to work or not after having the baby.

Talking to other working mums about their own situations can be very informative and helpful in your own decision making. Discuss your specific needs with your partner and family before coming to a decision.

What's happening to your baby?

✦ Your baby measures about 18cm from crown to rump (which is roughly half the size of a newborn baby) and weighs in the region of 450g. Her inherited characteristics from you and her father now begin to show, and whether she is smaller or larger than average becomes apparent from around this time.

✦ She is now swallowing more and more amniotic fluid on a regular basis. Her kidneys are processing this fluid, and she urinates regularly.

22

Your baby's body has begun to lay down fat under the skin, and his unique fingerprints are forming.

What's going on with you?

✦ By now you may well have developed a dark line (known as 'linea nigra') that runs from your belly button and down into your pubic hair. This is common in pregnant women, especially those with darker skin.

✦ Some pregnant women find that patches of skin on the face have changed colour. Usually, if you are dark-skinned, the patches (known as 'chloasma') are paler than your normal skin colour; if you are fair-skinned, they are darker. Most commonly, they occur on the cheeks, chin and nose, and disappear in the weeks following the birth.

What's happening to your baby?

✦ Your baby's hands are fully formed. The fingers will bend and stretch, and will grasp whatever they come into contact with. Often, this will be the umbilical cord.

✦ Hair is appearing on the scalp, and your baby now has eyelashes and also eyebrows.

✦ Although the fetus is still quite thin, his body is beginning to store fat. Over the coming weeks, he will lay down enough fat to give him the chubby look associated with healthy newborn babies. Fat helps to retain heat in the body; until he has enough fat on his frame to keep him warm enough, the hair that covers his skin now (known as 'lanugo') will do the job instead. This hair will disappear at around week 36, when the baby's body has enough fat on it to keep him warm.

✦ Your baby can hear your heartbeat, the noises made by your digestive system and the blood flowing through your blood vessels. He can also hear any louder sounds from outside your body.

"Ask your friends and family what items are most useful and what they don't think is necessary. Use their advice to help you plan your baby shopping. You'll need a lot less than you would expect."

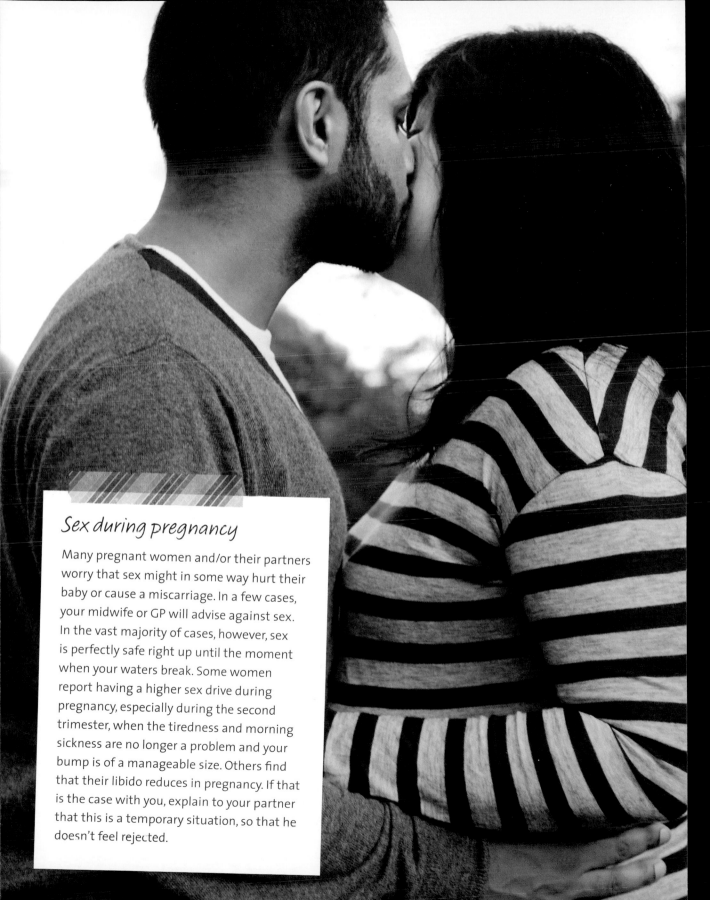

Sex during pregnancy

Many pregnant women and/or their partners worry that sex might in some way hurt their baby or cause a miscarriage. In a few cases, your midwife or GP will advise against sex. In the vast majority of cases, however, sex is perfectly safe right up until the moment when your waters break. Some women report having a higher sex drive during pregnancy, especially during the second trimester, when the tiredness and morning sickness are no longer a problem and your bump is of a manageable size. Others find that their libido reduces in pregnancy. If that is the case with you, explain to your partner that this is a temporary situation, so that he doesn't feel rejected.

23

> ✔ Make adjustments to your workspace to make yourself more comfortable, so that you can focus better on your work

You might be finding it difficult to stay focused at work these days as you become increasingly tuned in to your baby.

What's going on with you?

✦ You might find that you are less sharp in your thinking, more forgetful, a bit more absent-minded – baby brain has begun! However, baby brain can play havoc with your life because you find it more difficult to keep things organised. Ask for help if necessary. Simplify your life to make it easier, and write yourself notes as reminders for those really important things!

✦ It's important to do what you can to ensure your pregnancy does not affect your professional life. For instance, you may be finding it difficult to concentrate on your work right now. If your boss knows that you are pregnant, he or she might be looking out for signs that you are losing interest. Take every opportunity to show your dedication. Use your break times to rest and to invigorate yourself with some gentle exercise. Eat small amounts throughout the day to boost your energy, and drink plenty of water.

Carpal tunnel syndrome

If you experienced a tingling sensation, pins and needles, or numbness in your hands and fingers, see your GP or midwife, as you may have something called 'carpal tunnel syndrome'. Due to pregnancy hormones, nerves passing through the carpal tunnel (found in your wrist) become squeezed, which causes the symptoms. It might be helpful to wear a splint during the day and raise up your arm on a pillow at night. In the majority of cases, carpal tunnel syndrome disappears in the weeks or months immediately following the birth.

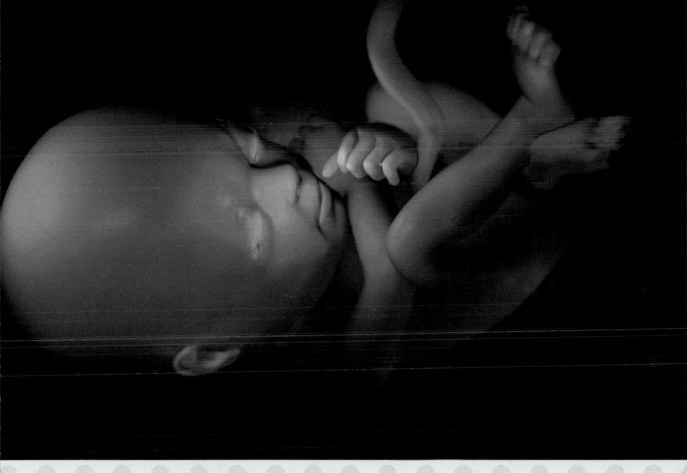

What's happening to your baby?

✦ Your baby's skin is still very thin, see-through and somewhat wrinkled. Her blood vessels are visible through her skin. This will change over the next few weeks as her body continues to lay down fat.

✦ She is now able to recognise your voice. Some fetuses at this stage move rhythmically to their mothers' voices or to music. You may feel silly talking to your baby, but it could help you to bond with her, and it will certainly get you into a habit of talking to her that continues after the birth. Research shows that the more you talk to young babies, the more quickly and effectively they learn to speak, so there's no harm in getting into this habit now. And if your baby readily recognises your voice after she is born, she may be comforted by it.

"If you are affected by carpal tunnel syndrome, be careful when lifting heavy items such as kettles and saucepans, especially in the mornings."

24

✔ If this is your first baby, read up on caring for newborn and young babies

Your baby's activity levels and routine might be becoming obvious to you at this stage, and you may find that he is most active at nighttime, just as you lie down to go to sleep!

What's going on with you?

◆ You may feel a strong bond with your baby and have nurturing and protective feelings towards him already. This mothering instinct, however, might not kick in until after the birth, so don't worry if you don't feel this way. It doesn't make you any less of a woman or a mother.

◆ It's likely that you've been able to feel your baby's movements for a while now, although some women are less able to feel the movements than others, especially if the placenta is located towards the front of the body. If you can feel the movements, you can work out when your baby is active or asleep. At this stage, your baby has lots of space in the womb, so he can make fairly large movements. As he becomes bigger, his space will become more restricted, and you will find that the types of movements he makes change, along with how often he moves.

Fluid retention

It is quite normal for hands, feet and ankles to become swollen during pregnancy as a result of fluid retention, a condition known as 'oedema'. Your midwife will assess the swelling at each check up to ensure that it is within the normal range. If you find you have any sudden and extreme swelling, see your GP or midwife immediately, as this could indicate pre-eclampsia, which is a very dangerous condition.

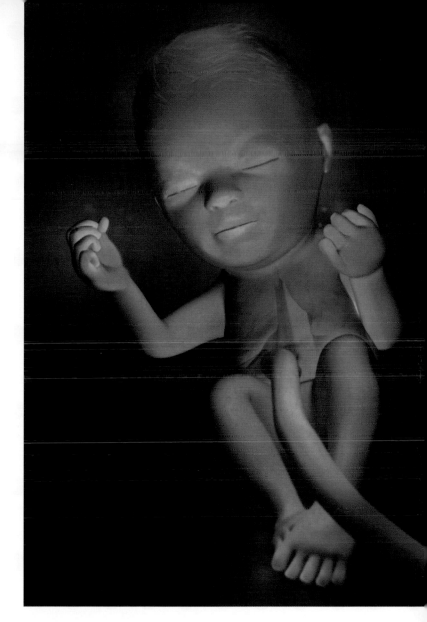

What's happening to your baby?

✦ Your baby measures 21cm from crown to rump and weighs roughly 630g.

✦ His lungs are filled with amniotic fluid, which is helping all the air vessels inside them to develop and grow.

✦ All his major organs are now fully developed.

✦ Your baby's eyelids have begun to open, and he is developing creases on his palms.

"Your antenatal visits will be more frequent from this point. Use the opportunity to ask your midwife for advice on things like late pregnancy, hospital bags, and so on, and to raise any concerns."

25

> ✓ Let your boss know this week in writing that you are pregnant

> ✓ Attend the next antenatal appointment this week

As your pregnancy progresses, it's likely that you will experience a few physical discomforts and changes. Don't worry – there are things that you can do to alleviate the problems.

What's going on with you?

✦ Over the next few weeks, you may find you suffer any of a range of physical problems associated with pregnancy, such as cramp (see page 77), sleep problems (see page 81) and digestive problems (see page 85). Ask your midwife for advice on coping strategies, and take heart – in most cases, the issue disappears once the baby is born.

✦ Due to your ever-increasing bump, you may experience back pain (see page 83). Maintain good posture when you are sitting or standing. You should also take care when bending down to pick up things that you do so safely and with as little strain on your back as possible.

What's happening to your baby?

✦ Your baby now hiccups and yawns regularly, both of which may help the development of her lungs.

✦ The effects of the period of intensive fat-storage over the past few weeks are visible, and your baby's arms and legs are becoming chubbier.

✦ Her head is still rather large in proportion to her body, but less so than it was before, and her proportions are approaching those of a newborn baby.

"Swimming is an excellent way of alleviating the aches and pains of pregnancy and staying in shape without stressing the ligaments and joints, which may be causing you discomfort."

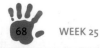

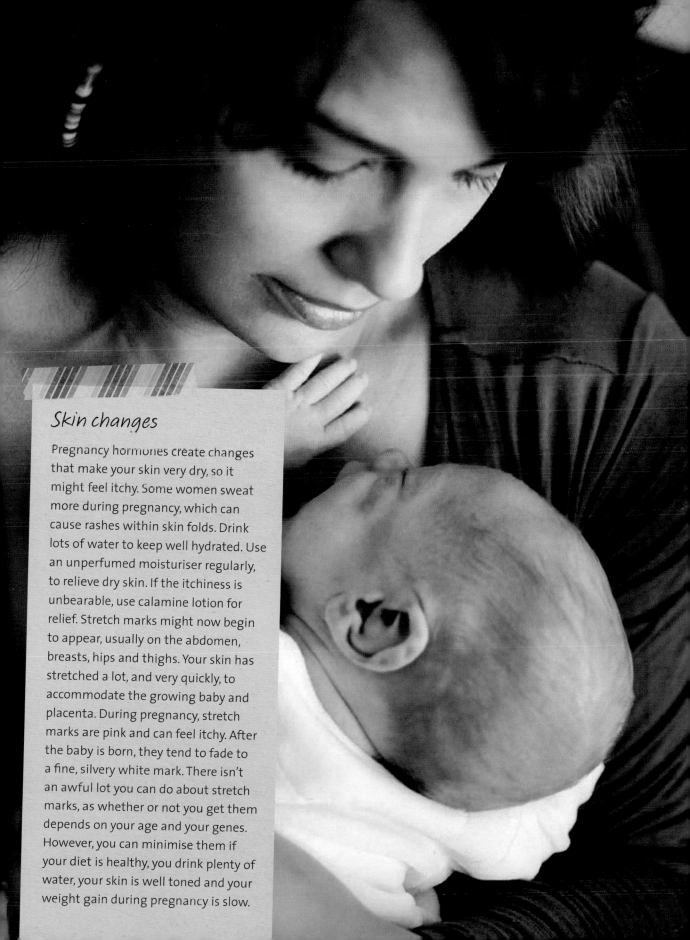

Skin changes

Pregnancy hormones create changes that make your skin very dry, so it might feel itchy. Some women sweat more during pregnancy, which can cause rashes within skin folds. Drink lots of water to keep well hydrated. Use an unperfumed moisturiser regularly, to relieve dry skin. If the itchiness is unbearable, use calamine lotion for relief. Stretch marks might now begin to appear, usually on the abdomen, breasts, hips and thighs. Your skin has stretched a lot, and very quickly, to accommodate the growing baby and placenta. During pregnancy, stretch marks are pink and can feel itchy. After the baby is born, they tend to fade to a fine, silvery white mark. There isn't an awful lot you can do about stretch marks, as whether or not you get them depends on your age and your genes. However, you can minimise them if your diet is healthy, you drink plenty of water, your skin is well toned and your weight gain during pregnancy is slow.

26

✓ Write a diet plan to help you stay in control of your weight gain

This is the last week of the second trimester. There's absolutely no hiding your pregnancy from people at this stage!

What's going on with you?

✦ Average weight gain during the second trimester is 0.5kg per week, around 6–6.5kg for the entire trimester. Your midwife will monitor your weight gain during pregnancy to check whether you are gaining too much or too little weight, and will advise you accordingly.

✦ Your bump is now sizeable, and you may experience heartburn and/ or indigestion, as the organs of your digestive system become more and more squashed.

What's happening to your baby?

✦ Your baby measures 23cm from crown to rump and weighs in the region of 800g.

✦ His coordination is improving, and his hand movements have become more precise.

✦ Your baby's fingernails are getting longer, and you may well find that they need to be cut not long after the birth to prevent scratches.

✦ His glands are already causing hormones that support his development to be released in his body.

✦ Although his body has been laying down fat, your baby is still very slender. The next trimester will see his body become significantly more rounded and 'bonny'.

"Reduce your sugar intake during pregnancy, as too much may cause gestational diabetes. This can lead to stillbirth, complications in labour and blood-sugar problems for the baby."

Supporting your pregnancy

At this stage of your pregnancy, your growing baby is well cushioned in a roomy womb, surrounded by plenty of amniotic fluid that conducts some of the sounds made by his mother's body and the outside world to his ears. The umbilical cord connects him to the placenta, which receives 400ml of blood per minute from the mother's bloodstream. This allows the placenta to pass on nutrients and oxygen to the baby, and return waste products from his body (see page 41). The mother's body also prevents some substances in her bloodstream that could be harmful to her baby from reaching the placenta and entering the baby's circulation. The womb is a thick wall of muscle that encases this world within the mother's body.

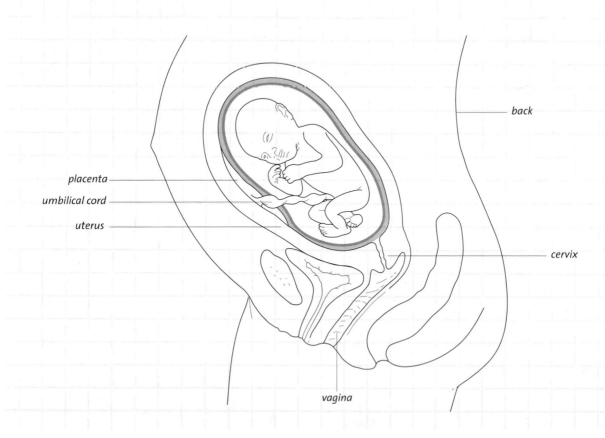

back

placenta

umbilical cord

uterus

cervix

vagina

27

- ✓ Review the list you have made of baby equipment

- ✓ Ask your friends which items from the list you can borrow from them

- ✓ Start fine-tuning your birth plan

During the last trimester of your pregnancy, your baby becomes a good deal larger and your body will feel the impact, but there are things you can do to alleviate discomforts. Knowing that you will soon hold your baby in your arms becomes more of an exciting reality.

What's going on with you?

✦ Make sure that your partner feels part of the pregnancy by discussing your antenatal appointments and sharing thoughts and feelings about the upcoming birth. It's easy for them to feel left out of this momentous event that's taking place in their parther's body, so find ways to keep your partner feeling involved.

✦ Is your partner intending to be at the birth with you? In many cases, the mother's partner, usually the father, attends the birth of the baby, but this isn't always so. This is a good time to establish whom your birth partner will be if you haven't thought about it already. Some women choose to have a female family member or close friend with them. Whomever you choose can begin to prepare themselves for the birth and attend antenatal classes with you.

What's happening to your baby?

✦ At the start of the third trimester, all of the baby's body systems are formed and established. They will now mature over the coming weeks.

✦ Your baby's brain is growing rapidly. So that it can fit inside the skull, the brain tissue folds over itself, and the fetal brain takes on the wrinkled and intricately folded look of a human brain.

✦ Her nervous system is maturing well, enabling her movements to become ever more sophisticated.

✦ There is still a good amount of space for your baby to move around inside the womb. Your body is currently producing less amniotic fluid than before, so she is less cushioned inside the womb. This makes it easier for you to feel her kicks and other movements than before.

"It's a good idea to plan to have someone with you when you give birth, to provide you with personal, emotional and practical support."

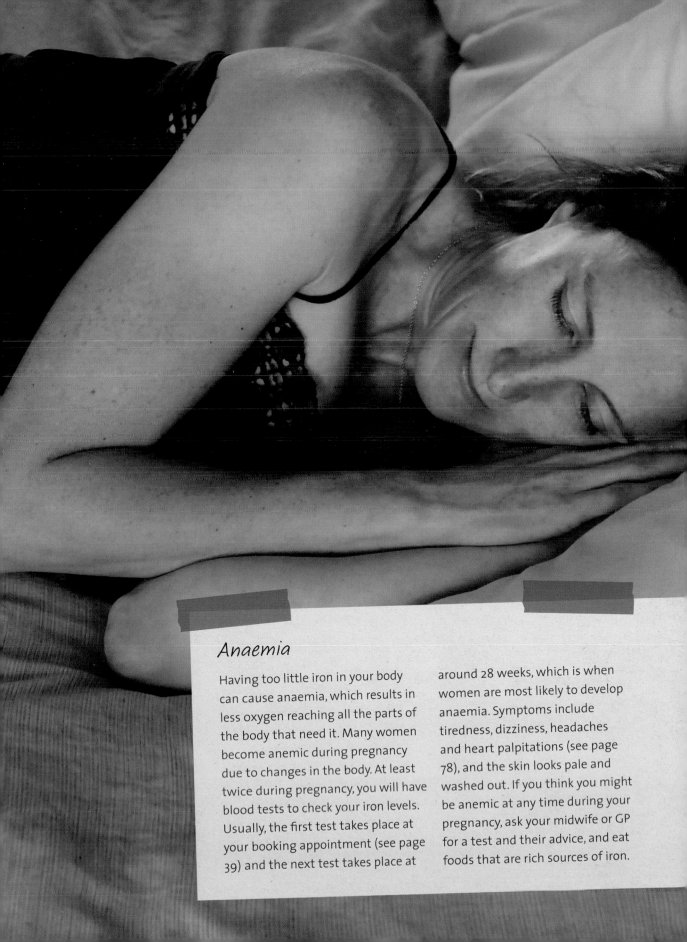

Anaemia

Having too little iron in your body can cause anaemia, which results in less oxygen reaching all the parts of the body that need it. Many women become anemic during pregnancy due to changes in the body. At least twice during pregnancy, you will have blood tests to check your iron levels. Usually, the first test takes place at your booking appointment (see page 39) and the next test takes place at around 28 weeks, which is when women are most likely to develop anaemia. Symptoms include tiredness, dizziness, headaches and heart palpitations (see page 78), and the skin looks pale and washed out. If you think you might be anemic at any time during your pregnancy, ask your midwife or GP for a test and their advice, and eat foods that are rich sources of iron.

28

✓ Attend the next antenatal appointment this week

✓ Have a urine test for anaemia and glycosuria

You may be hearing lots of advice about pregnancy and birth. Don't feel that you have to listen to it all. Change the subject if you feel the advice is not for you. Only you should be making choices about your pregnancy and the delivery, and you will feel empowered by doing so.

What's going on with you?

✦ Dealing with unwanted advice is something all pregnant women face at some point. The situation requires tact, as your loved ones may see your intention to do things differently as criticism of their choices. You'll need your friends around you at this time, so be open-minded, appreciate their experience, and be sensitive in your responses. Remember that there is no need to be defensive, as these are your decisions to make. Let them know that you appreciate their concern, but have thought through the issues carefully and chosen a course of action that's right for you.

✦ The lower part of your ribcage has now begun to arch outwards, to create more space for the growing womb. You might experience some pain in the lower ribs as a result, particularly if you are of a small build.

✦ It's common for women to experience heart palpitations during the third trimester (see page 78). They are nothing to be alarmed by even though they can feel highly uncomfortable.

What's happening to your baby?

✦ Your baby now measures 25cm from crown to rump and weighs roughly 1,000g.

✦ His eyes are now open and sensitive to light – if a strong light is shined on your tummy, he will turn away from it.

✦ The pattern of creases on his palms is now visible, and the toenails are forming, although they are not as well developed as the fingernails.

✦ Your baby has now laid down enough fat to smooth out some of the wrinkles on his skin.

"Often, parents, in-laws, friends or even your partner have an opinion on how things should be done, and may express their views in a way that makes you feel pressured to accept their advice. In such situations, you need tact and gentle firmness."

Gestational diabetes

Some women develop diabetes during pregnancy, which can cause complications for you and the baby. This condition can go unnoticed but is normally detected by the presence of glucose or sugar in your urine, which is tested by your midwife. If this is the case you'll be asked to have a glucose tolerance test to determine how your body deals with sugar. If the results fall outside the normal limits you will be diagnosed with gestational diabetes. Sometimes a change in diet and lifestyle is all that is needed but some women will need medication to bring their blood sugar under control. You will see an obstetrician who will teach you how to test your blood sugar, take your medication and help you make a plan for regular check ups.

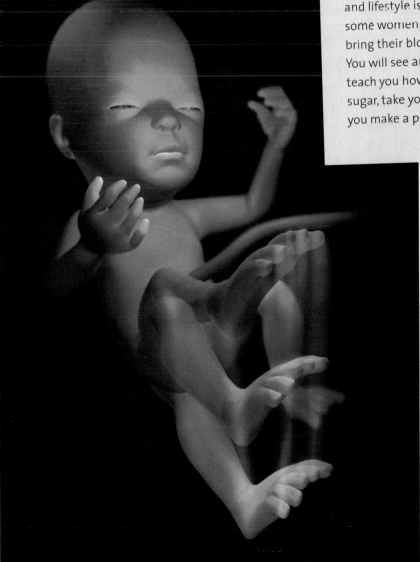

29

✓ Get out and about this week to take your mind off your pregnancy symptoms

You might be feeling fed up with your pregnancy by now. You've probably had too many conversations about deliveries and babies, and may be weary of your symptoms and feeling heavy. Don't worry – there's not long to go. Try to take your mind off the pregnancy for now.

What's going on with you?

✦ If you've had enough of the pregnancy for now, distract yourself with some social outings, your hobbies or a mini-break with your partner. Taking on a project at work might be just the thing to distract you from the aches and pains of pregnancy, and remind you that you are not just a baby machine, but also a woman with a full life.

✦ By now, the size of your growing bump will have altered your centre of gravity, and you might feel off balance. Also, pregnancy hormones have the effect of loosening your joints, making it more difficult to keep and regain your balance. In the vast majority of cases, a fall will cause absolutely no harm to the baby. If your blood type is 'rhesus negative', however, call your midwife for advice, as she may ask you to have an anti-D injection to prevent your body producing antibodies against rhesus positive blood (as the baby's blood type is still unknown).

What's happening to your baby?

✦ Your baby's lungs have been developing fast over the past few weeks and will continue to do so until the birth. From this week, her lungs have begun to produce a substance called 'surfactant', which aids your baby to exhale air after breathing in.

✦ Her bones are fully developed, but have not yet become hard.

"Try not to worry if you take a tumble – although you may have a few bumps and bruises, it's unlikely that your baby will be harmed, as she is well cushioned in the womb."

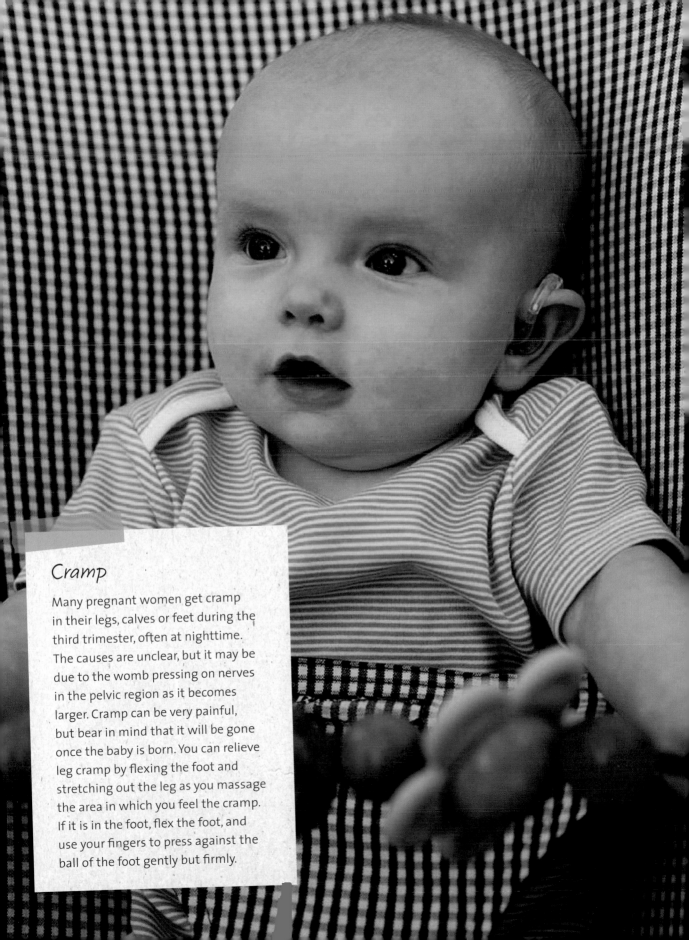

Cramp

Many pregnant women get cramp in their legs, calves or feet during the third trimester, often at nighttime. The causes are unclear, but it may be due to the womb pressing on nerves in the pelvic region as it becomes larger. Cramp can be very painful, but bear in mind that it will be gone once the baby is born. You can relieve leg cramp by flexing the foot and stretching out the leg as you massage the area in which you feel the cramp. If it is in the foot, flex the foot, and use your fingers to press against the ball of the foot gently but firmly.

30

✓ You qualify for Statutory Maternity Pay or Maternity Allowance this week

✓ If you haven't already done so, sign up to antenatal classes, as you should begin soon

What you eat can affect your baby's development. A diet rich in vitamins and minerals will give him the best start, as you will supply him with all the nutrients he needs for optimum growth. (See pages 12–17 for more information on diet during pregnancy.)

What's going on with you?

✦ You might be finding it difficult to breathe and frequently find yourself feeling short of breath. This is because the fundus (the top of the womb) is pressing up against the diaphragm, the muscle that controls your lungs breathing in and out. Also, the lungs themselves are compressed by the womb. If you feel light-headed or as if your breathing is too shallow, consciously take slow, deep breaths.

What's happening to your baby?

✦ Your baby measures 27cm from crown to rump and weighs in the region of 1,300g.

✦ His brain is developing rapidly. Each day, neurons (nerve cells) are forming in the brain. Eating oily fish, nuts and seeds, and plenty of protein will support this development.

✦ Eating a diet rich in iron will help your baby's body to produce the red blood cells that it needs.

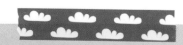

Heart palpitations

Roughly half of all pregnant women experience heart palpitations, most commonly during the third trimester. Although they can be frightening, it's important to note that they only rarely occur because of a serious condition. There are several possible causes. The heart has to work very hard during pregnancy, in order to pump more blood around the body, which can cause the palpitations. Anaemia (see page 73) can cause heart palpitations, as can stress and anxiety. If you experience heart palpitations with tightness in the chest and/or dizziness, contact your GP straight away.

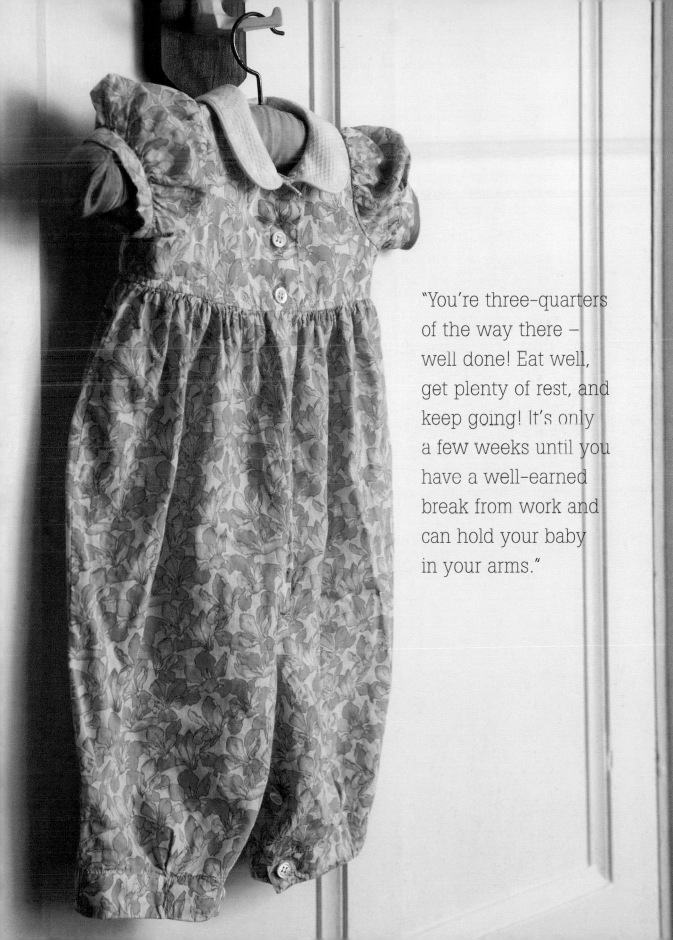

"You're three-quarters of the way there – well done! Eat well, get plenty of rest, and keep going! It's only a few weeks until you have a well-earned break from work and can hold your baby in your arms."

31

✓ Attend the next antenatal appointment this week

✓ Sign up to an antenatal aqua aerobics class this week

This is a good time to turn your attention to your baby's nursery. Perhaps you've been gathering a few items, borrowing others and planning how to put her room together. If, like some mothers, you feel a strong nesting instinct, harness it to prepare your home for your baby.

What's going on with you?

✦ The nesting instinct may have come home to roost by now. In the final few weeks of pregnancy, many women feel a strong urge to get the home clean and organised, ready for after the birth. If you experience this feeling, go with it. Use it to help you complete that unfinished DIY job or to decorate the nursery – or to organise your partner into doing it! Avoid climbing ladders and using decorating products containing substances that could be harmful to the baby. You could buy and arrange the baby's furniture, and make space for her clothes and other necessary items in her room. Consider where you will stash the pushchair and, in a few months, the highchair.

✦ Your breasts will be about 1kg heavier than they were before pregnancy. They begin to grow again around now as they prepare for breastfeeding and may leak a clear, orangey-yellow liquid (known as 'colostrum'). This is the type of milk that the breasts produce before the milk comes in on the third or fourth day after birth.

"You may want to get measured for nursing bras at this point. Factor in plenty of room for growth, as your breasts will still increase in size. Also, steer clear of underwired bras."

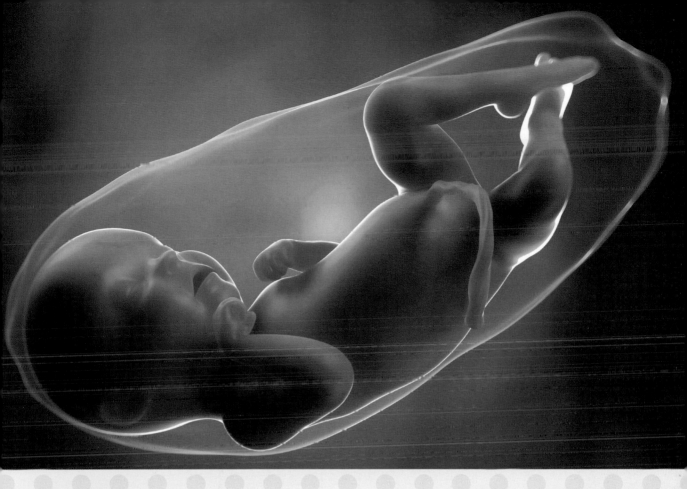

Sleeping comfortably

It can be difficult to find a comfortable sleeping position as the size of your bump increases during late pregnancy, and moving from one position to another becomes a major and cumbersome task. Few positions remain available to you, as it is bad for your circulation to lie on your back during later pregnancy, and you are no longer able to lie on your front. It might suit you to sleep on your side, with your uppermost leg bent and propped up on cushions, or with a cushion tucked between your knees. Use cushions to prop up your bump, too, if that feels comfortable. Some women prefer to sleep propped up in bed with a large V-shaped cushion.

What's happening to your baby?

✦ Much more fat is being laid down in your baby's body. Between weeks 28 and 31, she gained roughly 500g per week. Her skin has filled out and therefore looks less wrinkled, and her flesh is softer looking and more rounded. This new covering of fat makes the blood vessels less visible than they were before.

✦ Having gained a significant covering of fat in the recent weeks, your baby's body can now regulate its own temperature.

✦ The recent weight gain means that your baby no longer needs the hairy covering known as 'lanugo' across the skin (see page 62), and these hairs begin to thin out.

32

> ✔ *If you haven't done so already, buy the larger items of baby equipment, such as a cot*

By now, you may well have given the birth a good deal of thought and made notes for your birth plan. Now it's time to write it up, so that the midwives and obstetrician at the delivery are aware of your wishes.

What's going on with you?

✦ Your birth plan (see page 100–1) outlines the type of labour you wish to have. You don't need to write one to give birth; however, if you have strong feelings about what you would like to include or avoid, your birth plan is a place to express them. If you haven't already done so, it's a good idea to write yours up now, in case you go into labour early.

✦ It's very common to feel tired easily during this part of pregnancy. Finding it difficult to sleep can exacerbate the problem. Try to get as much rest as possible. If you have children and/or work, enlist the help of friends or family members when necessary. Your body needs good-quality rest in order to prepare for labour.

✦ Your belly button might now be protruding. It may even be visible through your clothing.

What's happening to your baby?

✦ Your baby now measures 28cm from crown to rump and weighs in the region of 1,700g.

✦ His eyes are now able to focus at a distance of roughly 15–20cm.

✦ This week marks the end of a four-week period of growth, starting at week 28, during which your baby's body laid down plenty of fat. He is now looking more substantial and plump, and his skin is smoother, the wrinkles having filled out a little.

✦ A quarter of all babies are in the breech position (see page 125) at this point. By the time your labour begins, however, the majority of these babies will have turned to the ideal head-down position.

"View your birth plan as a list of preferences, not a rigid plan, as things may not go as you wish. What's crucial is delivery of a well baby, as safely as possible, in the circumstances you find yourself on the day."

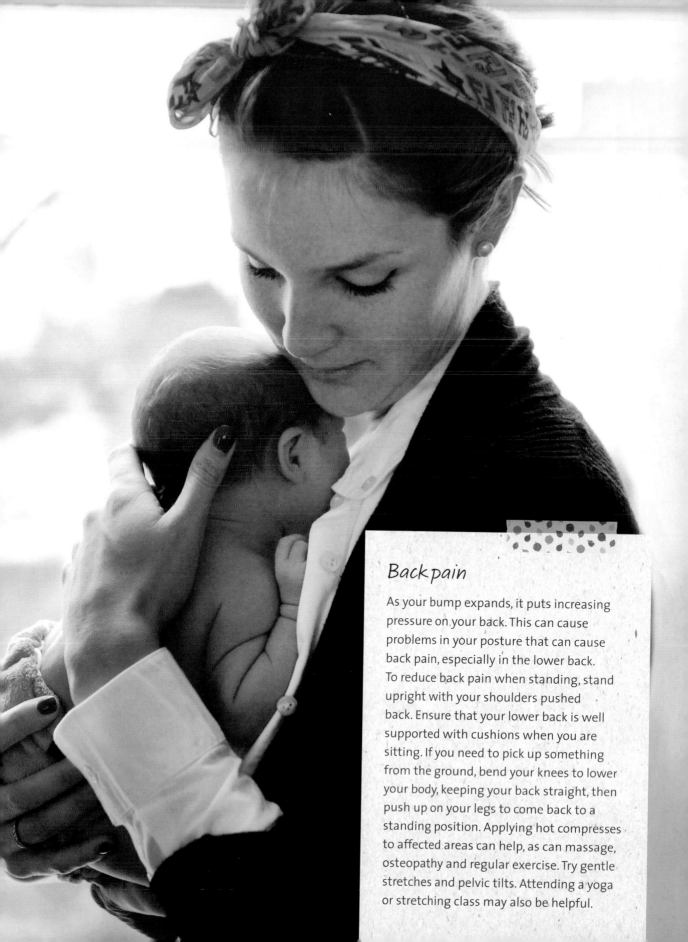

Back pain

As your bump expands, it puts increasing pressure on your back. This can cause problems in your posture that can cause back pain, especially in the lower back. To reduce back pain when standing, stand upright with your shoulders pushed back. Ensure that your lower back is well supported with cushions when you are sitting. If you need to pick up something from the ground, bend your knees to lower your body, keeping your back straight, then push up on your legs to come back to a standing position. Applying hot compresses to affected areas can help, as can massage, osteopathy and regular exercise. Try gentle stretches and pelvic tilts. Attending a yoga or stretching class may also be helpful.

33

✓ Remember to
practise pelvic-floor
exercises (see page 19)

As you inch towards the birth and life beyond it, your baby continues to reach milestones of development that are preparing her for life outside the womb.

What's going on with you?

✦ While the birth itself may be weighing heavy on your mind, no doubt you will have peeped beyond it to imagine what life will be like during your baby's first few months. It's difficult to know what to expect (see page 88), especially if this is your first baby. You might be wondering what your baby will be like, how you will feel when you hold her, what you'll need to learn to look after her and if your life after the birth will resemble your life before pregnancy in any way. Your feelings are likely to range from utter joy to petrified – sometimes within seconds! If you are the type of person who likes to know what to expect, it can be especially difficult to feel so out of control. Try to relax and go with it. Remember that being a mother is a natural process, and you are more than likely to find your way through it naturally.

What's happening to your baby?

✦ Your baby's brain and nervous system are now completely formed. Her lungs are still maturing, but a baby born at 33 weeks may need only a little help to breathe.

✦ Her bones are still hardening, using calcium from your diet, so make sure that you eat foods that are rich in calcium (see page 12–13).

"If you're a woman who likes a plan, it's difficult not knowing what to expect when the baby arrives. Try to relax and trust that your natural empathy towards your baby will guide you."

Digestive complaints

Pregnancy hormones can cause digestive problems in pregnancy. Eating small meals more frequently, avoiding rich and spicy foods, and eating your evening meal a minimum of two hours before you go to bed can all help to relieve digestive problems.

Heartburn and **indigestion** can be caused by the expanding womb pressing on the digestive organs. Try the following to alleviate your symptoms:

✦ take low-fat milk or probiotic natural yogurt either before or after you eat a meal, to neutralise the acid in your stomach
✦ raise up your head and shoulders when you sleep, using an extra pillow or two if necessary, to avoid reflux (the rise of gastric juices up the digestive tract)
✦ take an antacid medication that is suitable for pregnant women.

Constipation is common during pregnancy and can be caused by pregnancy hormones such as progesterone slowing down the digestive system. To avoid or eliminate constipation, try the following:

✦ eat plenty of fibre, found in wholegrain foods, fruits and vegetables
✦ drink less tea, coffee and colas – replace these with herbal teas and water
✦ ensure you drink 2–3 litres of fluids per day
✦ exercise regularly.

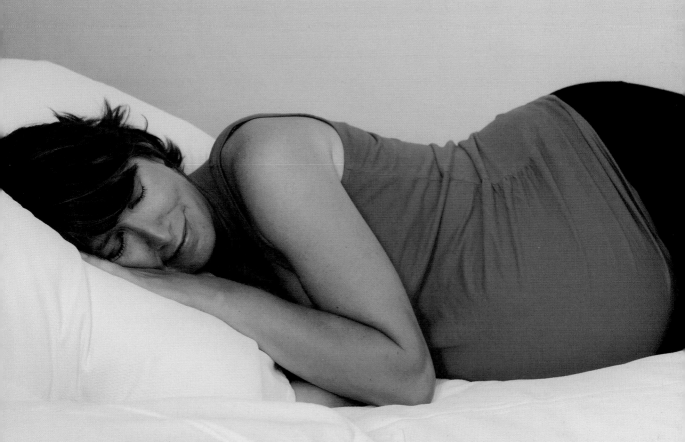

34

✓ Attend the next antenatal appointment this week

✓ Research baby monitors and buy one

Around about now, you might experience false contractions, known as Braxton Hicks contractions. Don't confuse them for the real thing! They are practice runs for your womb as your body prepares for birth.

What's going on with you?

✦ You may notice your womb becoming hard and tight at times. Braxton Hicks contractions usually begin at around week 34, although they can start in the second trimester, especially if you have had a baby before. See the box below for advice on how to distinguish Braxton Hicks from real contractions.

✦ If you find your bump and hips feel sore from walking, try wearing a pregnancy support band. This will help to alleviate lower back pain, too. If you don't feel comfortable wearing a support band, use your hands to support the weight of your bump as you walk.

Braxton Hicks contractions

Braxton Hicks contractions last for roughly 30–60 seconds, but can go on for as long as 2 minutes. They are sometimes called 'practice contractions' because the muscles of the womb tighten during Braxton Hicks contractions, which can be painful, especially as your due date approaches. It can be difficult to tell more intense Braxton Hicks contractions apart from real contractions. Unlike real contractions, however, Braxton Hicks do not become more intense or frequent over time, and will ease away and disappear. Also, they tend to feel uncomfortable rather than painful. Braxton Hicks can be triggered by a full bladder, sex, dehydration, your bump being touched, or you or the baby being more active than usual. If you are in discomfort, try walking around, changing your sitting position or relaxing using breathing techniques you learned in antenatal classes. Hot compresses or a warm bath may ease the discomfort. If you are unsure if you are having Braxton Hicks or the real thing, ask your midwife or one at the local maternity unit for advice.

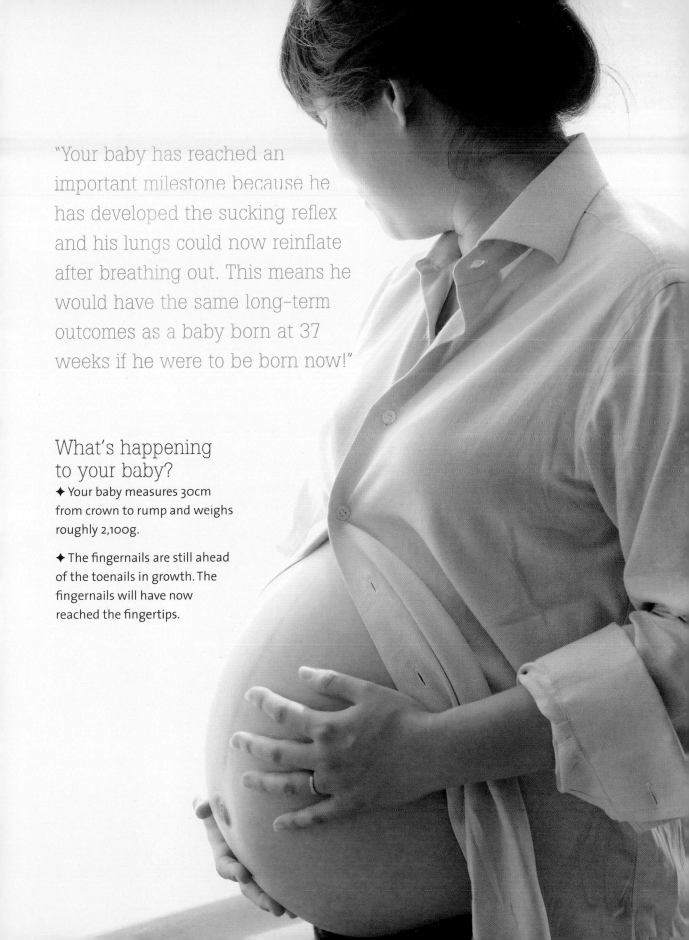

"Your baby has reached an important milestone because he has developed the sucking reflex and his lungs could now reinflate after breathing out. This means he would have the same long-term outcomes as a baby born at 37 weeks if he were to be born now!"

What's happening to your baby?

✦ Your baby measures 30cm from crown to rump and weighs roughly 2,100g.

✦ The fingernails are still ahead of the toenails in growth. The fingernails will have now reached the fingertips.

35

✓ Practise the breathing and relaxation techniques you have learned in your antenatal classes

✓ Buy new breastfeeding/ maternity bras

This is a good time to start thinking about what life will be like after the birth. If you don't have children already, it can be difficult to imagine what to expect.

What's going on with you?

✦ Preparing for life with a newborn baby can provide you with a good distraction from any anxieties you may feel about the labour itself. Ask other mums for their tips and advice, and select the strategies that sound most sensible to you. Think about how you will get out and about with your baby. Buy nappies, baby grows, cotton wool, muslins and other baby equipment, so that when the day comes for you to welcome your baby into your home you are fully prepared for her.

✦ The amount of blood flowing through your veins reaches an all-time high this week – you have more than 45 per cent greater volume of blood than before pregnancy. This causes your blood pressure to increase slightly over the coming weeks as you approach labour. You are likely to feel more hot and sweaty, too, as the extra blood volume makes your body warmer.

✦ Increased blood volume can cause swelling and puffiness in your hands and feet, known as oedema (see page 66). Try flexing and pointing your feet repeatedly, and rotating your foot in circles in both directions. Drink lots of water, and exercise gently to improve your circulation. Make sure you are wearing comfortable shoes, and avoid standing up for long periods of time. If the swelling is sudden, contact your GP or midwife as this could be a sign of pre-eclampsia, which is very dangerous for both you and the baby if it is not treated promptly.

"It's a good idea to practise buckling your baby's car seat using a teddy or doll, so that the journey home with your newborn baby is less stressful and more exciting."

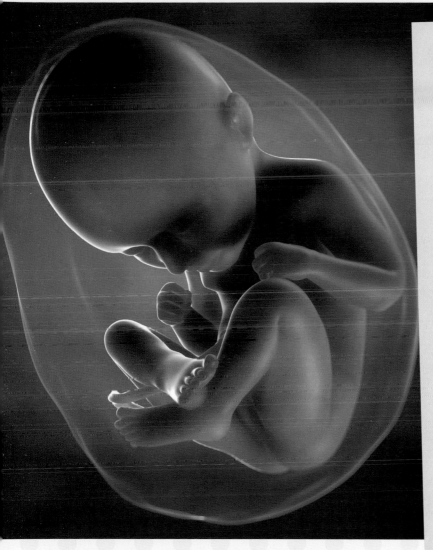

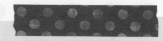

Preparing your hospital bag

You'll need to get a bag together that contains the things you'll need to help you through the birth. It's sensible to prepare the bag now, in case you go into labour early. Even if you are planning for a home birth, you should pack a hospital bag just in case you suddenly need to go to the hospital. It's a good idea to pack two bags – one containing items for the birth and one with things for after the birth. Useful items for your labour bag might include: a nightdress or large T-shirt, dressing gown, slippers and socks; a towel and flannel; water bottles, cartons of juice with straws, and snacks; massage oil; TENS machine; birthing ball or birthing stool; camera; music system and/or a book. Useful items for your post-labour bag might include: a clean nightdress, toiletries, maternity bras and breast pads, sanitary towels and disposable underwear; maternity clothes; baby clothes (a few sleepsuits, vests, a hat, and warmer outer clothes); disposable nappies, cotton wool, barrier cream; ear plugs and eye mask.

What's happening to your baby?
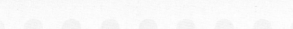

✦ The baby's digestive system is now fully functional, ready for life after birth.

✦ Your baby's body continues to lay down fat, but there is not yet enough fat on her body to keep her warm if she were to be born early. (Premature babies usually need to be kept in an incubator for a little while.)

✦ The level of amniotic fluid is at its maximum this week. Over the coming weeks, the amount will slowly reduce.

36

✓ Attend the next antenatal appointment this week

✓ Stock up the freezer with batches of home-cooked meals or ready meals in preparation for the first couple of weeks after the birth

In preparation for the birth, your baby's head might 'engage' as early as this week. This means that the baby's head has begun to move down into the pelvic cavity, towards the exit!

What's going on with you?

✦ When the baby's head engages, your bump will suddenly seem lower on your torso than it was. As the womb moves downwards, it presses down more heavily on the bladder, so you might need to pee more often. The pressure, however, on your lungs and digestive organs is likely to reduce, so you'll be able to breathe more easily, your appetite will return to normal and any symptoms of digestion problems will improve. If this is your first pregnancy and the head has not engaged, the midwife might arrange for a scan to establish the reason. Common reasons for failure to engage include: a fibroid in your womb; your baby is in a breech position (see page 125) or placenta praevia (in which the placenta is low in the womb). Don't worry if the baby's head hasn't engaged – in many instances, it doesn't happen until labour begins. Also, it is less likely to engage if you have had a baby before.

What's happening to your baby?

✦ The baby has now developed the ability to make all the sucking movements he needs in order to be able to feed when he is born.

✦ If your baby were to be born prematurely now, he may not need to stay in the neonatal unit but will need his blood sugar and temperature monitored regularly.

"If your placenta was 'low' at your 20-week scan, you will have a repeat scan this week to check that it does not cover or partially cover the cervix."

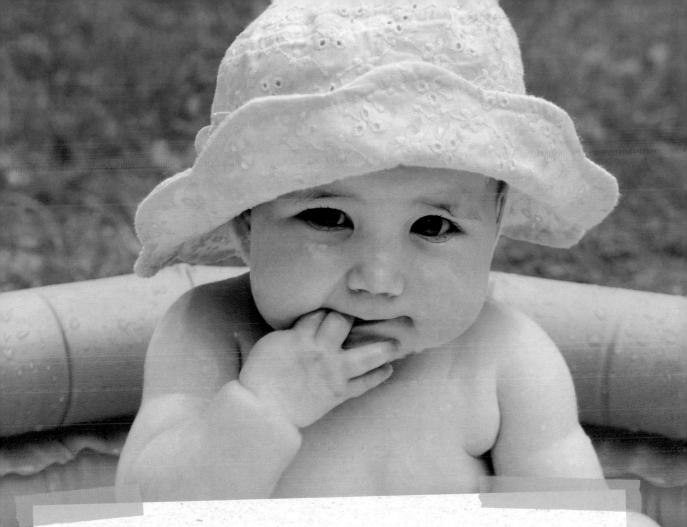

Embarrassing complaints

These two unpleasant conditions are very commonly experienced by women during the third trimester.

Haemorrhoids (piles) are simply varicose veins around the outside or in the opening of the anus. As you approach the end of pregnancy, the weight of the womb pressing down on the pelvis can prevent blood flowing back to the heart, causing piles. They can be painful and itchy, and result in bleeding from the rectum. There is no cure for piles, but in most cases they disappear once the baby is born. To alleviate the symptoms, try the following:

✦ avoid lifting heavy items
✦ try not to become constipated (see page 85), which can exacerbate piles

✦ practise pelvic-floor exercises (see page 19)
✦ apply an ice pack to the area for a few minutes to reduce inflammation
✦ apply over-the-counter haemorrhoid cream or ointment.

Stress incontinence describes the condition in which a little urine unexpectedly escapes from your bladder when you sneeze, cough or laugh. This happens because of the weight of the womb pressing down on the pelvic-floor muscles. They receive a further battering during labour. Practising pelvic-floor exercises will strengthen pelvic-floor muscles and help to reduce or avoid the problem. Use a sanitary towel to help keep yourself fresh and clean.

37

✓ Make a list of important telephone numbers that may be useful during labour, such as those for the midwife, labour ward, GP surgery and a local taxi firm

✓ Use a waterproof sheet to protect your mattress in case your waters break when you are in bed

This week, you are considered to be 'at term' and, if your baby were to be born now, she would be considered to be an early rather than a premature baby.

What's going on with you?

✦ You are probably getting fed up with having to make frequent trips to the loo at nighttime. If you find that your sleep is disturbed, try not to drink too many liquids in the evenings, but make sure that you drink plenty of fluids during the day to stay well hydrated.

What's happening to your baby?

✦ The space available to your baby in which to move around reduces bit by bit as she grows. You will still be able to notice her larger movements easily, but you will find her smaller movements less easy to feel.

✦ Your baby now has a firm grasp, as you will soon find out!

✦ She will now turn her head towards a light source.

"Your baby's movements are your only indication of her well-being, so note how they have changed now that there is less room for her to move. If there is a change in her pattern of movements, let your midwife know immediately, so that the baby's heartbeat can be monitored for reassurance."

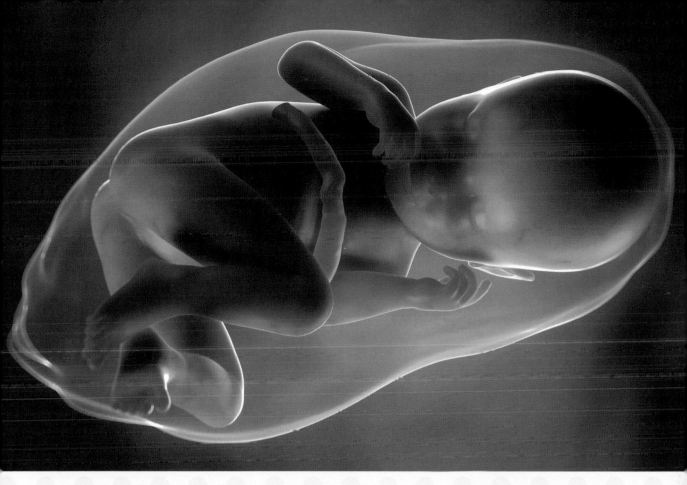

Varicose veins

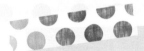

Varicose veins are very common in the third trimester and are caused by the changes to the circulatory system during pregnancy. They tend to come up on the legs and also around the anus (see box on Haemorrhoids, page 91); in most cases, they reduce or disappear once the baby is born. If you have developed varicose veins during the third trimester, try the following:

✦ avoid standing up for long periods. Particularly, avoid standing still. Move around on your feet as much as you can

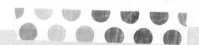

✦ keep your legs raised whenever you are sitting down

✦ exercise frequently to keep your circulation moving

✦ use pregnancy support tights and, ideally, put them on while you are still in bed in the morning. This will prevent the veins from dilating too much once you stand up. One in ten women will develop varicose veins on the vulva during pregnancy. They tend not to cause problems during labour and usually disappear after the birth.

38

✓ Attend the next antenatal appointment this week

✓ Keep your hand-held notes nearby at all times, and remember to take them with you whenever you go out

✓ Go swimming

Your baby is now ready to be born, and you could go into labour at any time, although it's unlikely to happen this week if this is your first pregnancy. Moving around may feel like hard work, and sleeping may now be a very uncomfortable experience.

What's going on with you?

✦ Your womb weighed only 50–60g before pregnancy, compared with the 1,000g it roughly weighs now. Your bump might extend to roughly 18cm above your belly button. You might feel like a beached whale when you lay down and feel as if you need a crane to lift you up to standing. Your body is working hard to keep your term-size baby alive and well, so get plenty of rest. Your body also needs to be well rested for labour.

✦ Prepare yourself mentally for labour. Remind yourself of the birthing positions and breathing exercises you learned in antenatal classes. Read up on the three stages of labour (see pages 106–19) so that you know what to expect. Familiarise yourself with how labour may begin (see page 104–5). If you're still at work, it may be wise to begin your maternity leave now, so that you can focus your energies on the upcoming birth.

What's happening to your baby?

✦ Your baby now measures roughly 34cm from crown to rump and weighs about 3,000g.

✦ Although his lungs are mature enough for him to breathe on his own if he were to be born now, the air passages will continue to develop after birth as they are not yet as formed as they would be at 40 weeks.

✦ Your baby's toenails now reach the ends of his toes. The covering of fine hair (lanugo, see page 62) has almost completely disappeared.

✦ His skull bones are now fully developed, but they are not yet joined together and they have not yet hardened. This is so that they can slide over one another during the birth, in order for the head to be able to take on a shape that is easier to pass through the birth canal.

Supporting your baby

The placenta is still supplying all your baby's nutritional and oxygen requirements. This amazing organ, grown especially to nurture your baby, is now fully mature and will no longer continue to grow. It is about 2–3cm thick, roughly 25cm in diameter and weighs 500–700g.

Right now, the placenta is at its most efficient, but from this point onwards, until the birth, its stores of nutrients will be used up, so that nothing is wasted by this highly efficient organ.

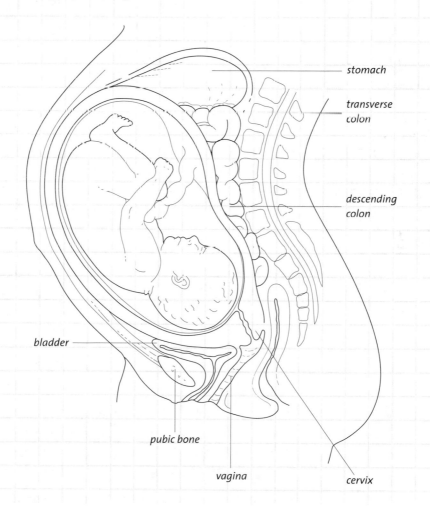

stomach

transverse colon

descending colon

bladder

pubic bone

vagina

cervix

"Enjoy your carefree days while you still have them. Catch up with friends and family, and enjoy meals out – it could be a while before you can do so again, with a newborn in tow!"

39

✔ *Treat yourself to a haircut or some beauty treatments while you still have the time*

✔ *Buy newborn-size nappies in preparation for your baby*

Your baby's patterns of movement are probably quite familiar to you by now. Keep a mental note of any changes from the norm, and report anything significant to your midwife, particularly if you feel her moving less often than usual.

What's going on with you?

✦ Your baby now has a lot less room to manouevre in the womb. Mothers tend to feel movements most often during the afternoons and evenings at this stage of pregnancy. Notice when your baby is still for a long time – this is when she is asleep. Periods of sleep often last for 20–40 minutes and rarely for more than 90 minutes. If you feel there has been a significant change in your baby's sleep and wakefulness pattern, contact your midwife, who will advise you. Although it is statistically unlikely that there will be a problem with the baby, it is good to rule out any serious problems, such as a lack of oxygen to the baby.

✦ You might be feeling anxious, impatient and nervous about the birth at this stage. Try to rest and keep your mind occupied. Go swimming, take naps on the sofa, read a book, cook some meals for the freezer, meet up with friends or family. Make sure that you don't undertake any heavy tasks; instead, try to prepare mentally for the birth. Keep calm and carry on! You will have your baby in your arms soon.

What's happening to your baby?

✦ Your baby measures 50cm from crown to rump and weighs roughly 3,000–3,500g.

✦ She has been swallowing amniotic fluid, which now contains a few waste products. Her body transforms these into a waste substance called 'meconium', which is stored in her colon, ready to be passed as a stool once she is born.

✦ The baby now makes regular breathing movements in preparation for using her lungs to breathe for the first time when she is born.

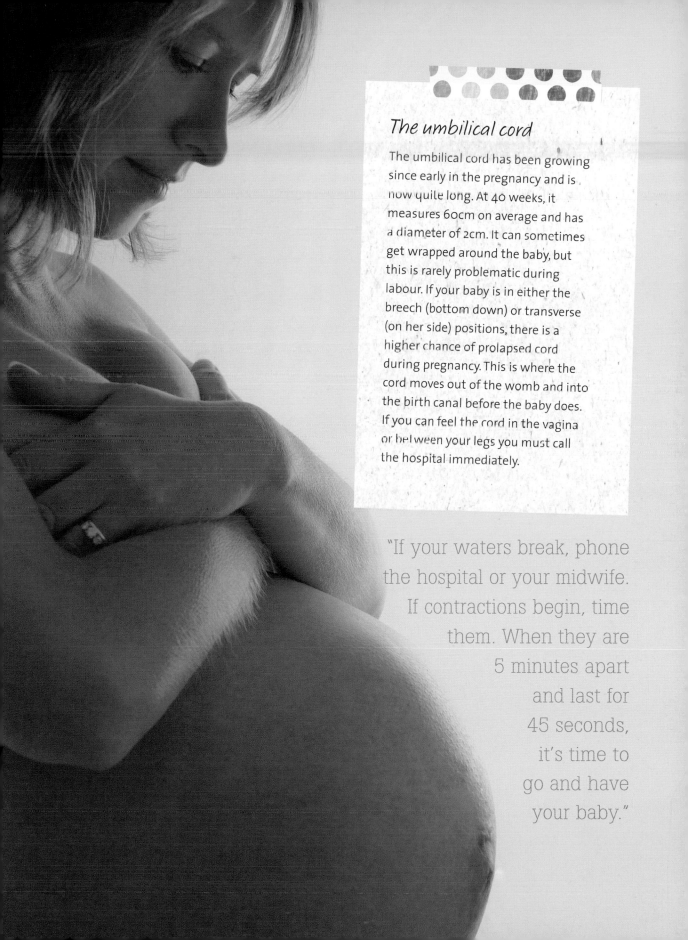

The umbilical cord

The umbilical cord has been growing since early in the pregnancy and is now quite long. At 40 weeks, it measures 60cm on average and has a diameter of 2cm. It can sometimes get wrapped around the baby, but this is rarely problematic during labour. If your baby is in either the breech (bottom down) or transverse (on her side) positions, there is a higher chance of prolapsed cord during pregnancy. This is where the cord moves out of the womb and into the birth canal before the baby does. If you can feel the cord in the vagina or between your legs you must call the hospital immediately.

"If your waters break, phone the hospital or your midwife. If contractions begin, time them. When they are 5 minutes apart and last for 45 seconds, it's time to go and have your baby."

40

✔ Attend the next antenatal appointment. If you are still pregnant next week, you will have one then, too

✔ Keep active – take gentle walks and go swimming

You're finally at 40 weeks. Very soon, you'll be holding your baby. Being overdue is common, particularly if this is your first pregnancy, so you may have to wait just a little bit longer.

What's going on with you?

✦ Very few babies arrive on their due date, but once you have passed the due date the pregnancy is considered 'overdue' (see box, opposite). You may well be feeling impatient for the birth now and tired of being on red alert at all times. Being heavily pregnant can be exhausting, especially if you go far past your due date. Get plenty of rest.

✦ Your skin has had to stretch a whopping 70–150cm in order to accommodate the extra bulk around your body during pregnancy. Amazingly, the skin will all shrink back to its pre-pregnancy condition in the weeks after the birth.

What's happening to your baby?

✦ The baby measures 36cm from crown to rump and weighs approximately 3,400g. His total body length is roughly 50cm.

✦ His fingernails have grown enough to extend past the fingertips.

✦ If your baby is caucasian, he will have blue eyes. If your baby is African or Asian, his eyes will be dark grey or light brown. They will remain this colour for a few months after the birth, before taking on the eye colour that your baby has genetically inherited.

"You may experience a 'show' (see page 104) soon before labour, or after a vaginal stretch and sweep. It's completely normal, but if it contains more blood than mucus, contact your midwife."

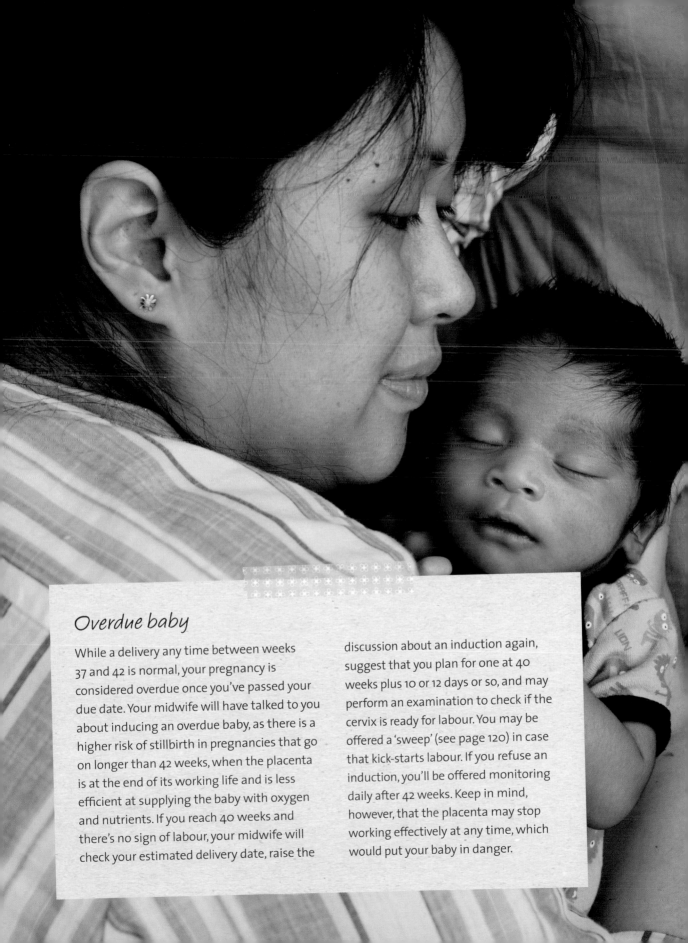

Overdue baby

While a delivery any time between weeks 37 and 42 is normal, your pregnancy is considered overdue once you've passed your due date. Your midwife will have talked to you about inducing an overdue baby, as there is a higher risk of stillbirth in pregnancies that go on longer than 42 weeks, when the placenta is at the end of its working life and is less efficient at supplying the baby with oxygen and nutrients. If you reach 40 weeks and there's no sign of labour, your midwife will check your estimated delivery date, raise the discussion about an induction again, suggest that you plan for one at 40 weeks plus 10 or 12 days or so, and may perform an examination to check if the cervix is ready for labour. You may be offered a 'sweep' (see page 120) in case that kick-starts labour. If you refuse an induction, you'll be offered monitoring daily after 42 weeks. Keep in mind, however, that the placenta may stop working effectively at any time, which would put your baby in danger.

Birth and your first few hours

Women have been giving birth for millenia, so remember that you are about to do something that comes naturally. A little knowledge can help you to relax when the big day comes, as you'll have the confidence of knowing you're as prepared as you can be.

Writing a Birth Plan

A birth plan allows you to outline your preferences for labour and birth. It's not necessary to have one, but the process of writing one allows you to consider your preferences. It will also present an opportunity to discuss your choices with your healthcare professionals and help them to tailor your birth to suit you.

Informing yourself

If you choose to write a birth plan, first learn everything you can about labour and birth (see pages 104–130), including Caesarean sections (which account for 25–30 per cent of births in the UK) and assisted deliveries. This way you can make informed and realistic decisions before writing down your wishes.

When you come to write your birth plan, make sure that you cover the important things, such as who your birth partner will be, what type of atmosphere you want in the room in which you give birth, your preferences for pain-relief methods, whether your partner intends

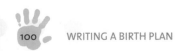

Birth partners

Your birth partner's role is to support you during labour and birth. Many women choose their life partner, but this isn't the best choice for every couple. Some women prefer a female friend or family member. Others have both – most hospitals will allow you to have up to two people with you. Choose your birth partner(s) wisely. Their role is to encourage you throughout the process, remaining sensitive to your needs; to see to your practical needs, providing you with massages, snacks or sips of water as necessary; to maintain an atmosphere of peace in which you can deliver your baby; and to communicate with medical staff on your behalf when you feel unable to do so. They must be able to keep calm when things become stressful, and able to be assertive with medical staff when necessary, without becoming aggressive. They need to understand that things can change quickly and plans may need to be dropped in order to protect mother and baby. They must be able to ask questions in order to understand what is going on, and be ready to step back when you don't want their help.

Your birth partner should read up on labour and birth, including Caesarean section and assisted deliveries, and familiarise themselves with your birth plan so they can ensure the staff know your preferences if necessary. Discuss with them in advance what type of support you feel you would like on the day, so that when the big day comes you feel you are working as a team.

to cut the umbilical cord, and if you would like an injection to manage the delivery of your placenta actively (see pages 114–15). You can also add details such as if you would like to give birth in a birthing pool (if the hospital staff/midwives allow this), the positions you would prefer for labour, and any alternative therapies you would like to use. Talking through your birth plan with your midwife before birth will allow you to discover whether any of your wishes go against hospital policy, so that you can adjust your plan accordingly.

It's important to remember that things might not go according to plan, and to prepare yourself for the unexpected. Remember, it's not your aim to 'get it right' and 'prove yourself'. Your aim as a mother is to deliver a healthy baby as safely as possible, and in order to do so it's best to remain open-minded so that you are able to respond to any situation as it arises. It is impossible to predict how things will go, so prepare yourself to go with the flow and not to be disappointed if things don't progress according to your plan. Even if you've given birth before, there is no guarantee that you will have the same type of delivery this time. Each birth is different. The hospital staff or homebirth midwives will do what they can to respect your wishes, but try to be ready to work with them to deliver your baby safely if things don't turn out exactly as you had hoped. It can still be a very positive experience.

Your Baby's Position

Your midwife or GP will begin to assess your baby's position within the womb from around the thirtieth week of pregnancy. Your baby's position can determine how your baby is delivered, and is assessed in four ways: the lie, presentation, position and engagement.

Lie

This refers to how your baby's body is lying within the womb. She could be positioned vertically (longitudinal), sideways/horizontally (transverse), or diagonally (oblique). At 37–40 weeks, 99 per cent of babies are positioned vertically, with either the head or the bottom close to the cervix. The transverse and oblique positions account for the remaining 1 per cent, and these babies will be delivered in the hospital by Caesarean section. Babies can change position right up until the last minute.

Presentation

This refers to the part of your baby that's closest to the cervix. It will be the first part of the baby's body to be delivered, so will 'present' itself first. In the vertical (longitudinal) lie, 95 per cent of babies are in the head-down position, or cephalic presentation. Breech presentation (with the feet closest to the cervix) accounts for the rest. Breech presentation is more common in premature babies and in second or subsequent deliveries.

Position

A baby in a vertical position with the head down may face different directions. Her back and the back of her head (the occiput) can face the back (posterior) of the mother's body, and she will usually also be facing towards the mother's side (lateral) – either her left or right. The exact position is noted, as some cephalic presentations take longer to deliver.

The ideal position is with the baby's back facing the front of the mother (OA). A baby in the OP position, with her back against the mother's back, takes longer to deliver because the widest part of the head is presenting, and the cervix dilates more slowly with the baby in this position. Also, the baby seems to descend through the birth canal more slowly when in OP. OP and occipital transverse (OT) positions can be extremely difficult to

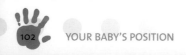

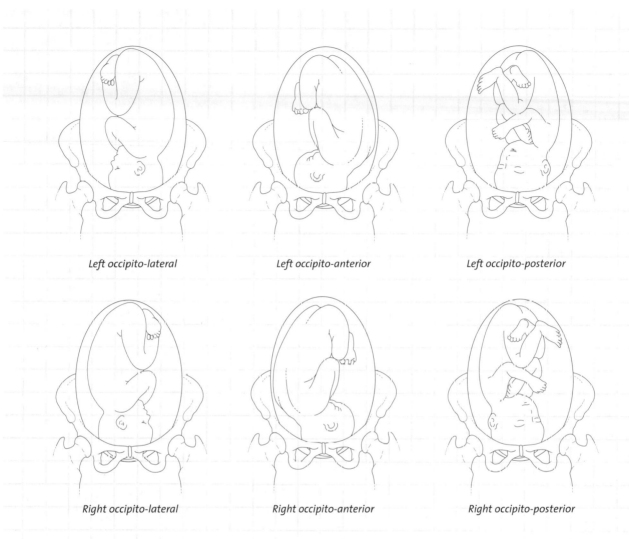

Left occipito-lateral   *Left occipito-anterior*   *Left occipito-posterior*

Right occipito-lateral   *Right occipito-anterior*   *Right occipito-posterior*

deliver, even if the mother has had a vaginal delivery before; rotation and delivery with forceps may be needed. Mothers are advised to stay upright and mobile during labour, as this encourages optimal fetal positioning and so a normal rate of progress in terms of labour and delivery, which is better for the baby than a long, drawn-out process.

Engagement

As your body prepares for birth, the baby's head moves down in the pelvis until it's in the correct position for birth. This process may begin at around 36 weeks in first pregnancies, later in subsequent ones. In the last month, your midwife will feel (palpate) the baby's head through your abdomen to assess engagement. There are levels of engagement, and the level your baby has reached will be recorded in your notes. When over half of the baby's head has dropped into the pelvic cavity, it is considered engaged.

Are You in Labour?

Labour is unpredictable, so it can be difficult to know when yours has begun. There are, however, a few signs. Essentially, it is the presence of regular contractions, which become stronger and stronger, that firmly marks the onset of labour.

Signs that labour is about to begin

There are three signs that women experience at the onset of labour, but not all women experience all or even any of them. Each labour is different, so things may not happen as they did in a previous labour. These signs don't come in any particular order, or guarantee that labour is about to begin! If you experience any of the below, it is likely that things are starting. A sign that labour has begun is that your cervix is dilating, but you will need a midwife to perform an internal examination to confirm it.

More Braxton Hicks

As labour nears, many women have more Braxton Hicks contractions (see page 86), which seem to become more intense, to the point that many first-time mothers believe that they are the real thing! Braxton Hicks contractions won't happen as often as real contractions – two per hour at the most. Nor do they get stronger or fade slowly, like real contractions. Another way of telling them apart is that if you can talk through the tightening, it's more than likely to be a Braxton Hicks contraction.

The 'show'

During pregnancy, the cervix has been 'plugged' by a lump of mucus that blocks bacteria from the womb. As the body prepares for labour, the cervix changes shape, which dislodges the plug. The blood-stained mucus or 'show' then comes out. Having a show does not guarantee that labour is about to begin, but it does show the body is preparing for labour.

Waters breaking

Also known as 'rupture of the membranes', this is when the amniotic sac surrounding your baby breaks, and amniotic fluid starts to leak out through the cervix. Usually, it is caused by the baby's head pressing down on the dilating cervix (see page 107) once contractions have begun. In 15 per cent of pregnancies, however, the waters break before contractions have begun.

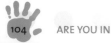

In some cases, there is a good deal of water, making it obvious that the waters have broken. In other cases, there is simply a trickle, which can be mistaken for leaking urine, a common side effect of late pregnancy (see page 91). To tell the difference, bear in mind that amniotic fluid is clear and has no smell, and it will continue to leak whenever you move.

Once your waters break

You need to let your midwife know if your waters have broken as you will need to be checked within the next six hours if your contractions haven't begun. If you have planned for a home birth, the midwife will come to you to check you. If you've booked a hospital birth, the midwife will ask you to go into the hospital for a check. Don't forget to take your hand-held notes with you, and it might be a good idea to grab a drink and a snack, as you can't predict how long you might be there.

The midwife can check if your waters have broken by inserting a plastic speculum into the vagina, to see if fluid can be seen pooling near the cervix. This is important because, if the waters have been broken for some time, there is a risk of infection in both the mother and baby.

The midwife may advise you to go home/stay at home and wait for labour to progress. Remember that, once your waters have broken, bacteria can enter the womb and cause damage to the baby. Make sure that, when you go to the toilet, you wipe yourself in a direction that moves away from the vaginal opening. This is particularly important if you are cleaning up after a bowel movement because fecal contamination is a very common cause of vaginal infection. Also, avoid sexual intercourse.

Labour commences within 24 hours of the waters breaking in 83 per cent of women. If, after a day, you haven't gone into labour, it is likely that your obstetrician will advise you to have your labour induced (if you are beyond 34 weeks), to reduce the risk of infection to your baby.

The start of contractions

You'll know labour is beginning when your contractions begin to come regularly. They increase in intensity, then fade away. If you have begun to feel contractions and think they are the real thing, note down both the length of each contraction and how long it takes from the start of one contraction to the start of the next. (Your birth partner could do this for you.) See if you can spot a timing pattern. Particularly in early labour, contractions can become frequent and intense, then ease off again. This is normal and nothing to worry about, so take advantage of the break.

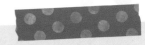

Meconium

If, when your waters break, you find that the amniotic fluid has a brown or green tinge to it, you must get to the hospital to be checked urgently, as the colour suggests that meconium is present in the amniotic fluid. Meconium is, you could say, your baby's first poo – it is the by-product his digestive system makes from the amniotic fluid he has ingested over time, which has bits of lanugo (see page 62), urine and other things in it. Usually, the baby will pass meconium after the birth. In some instances, he can pass the meconium while still in the womb, which may be very thick in the amniotic fluid or very diluted. Either type can leave him vulnerable to infection. If it is present, it is safest for your baby to be delivered as soon as possible.

The First Stage of Labour

Usually the longest stage of labour, the first stage sees your contractions slowly increase in intensity and frequency. There are three phases in this stage: the early phase, the active phase and the transition phase.

TENS machine

Transcutaneous Electronic Nerve Stimulation involves strapping four electrodes onto your back that are attached to an electronic (battery-operated) device that produces a gentle electrical current. When the current passes into your body via the electrodes, it interrupts the pain signals that the brain receives. In this way, TENS is frequently used by labouring women for pain relief. The current does not affect the baby, and you can control the device to produce the current once a contraction begins.

Monitoring your progress

During the first stage, your midwife will regularly monitor your baby's heart rate to ensure that all is well. In order to monitor your progress through this stage of your labour, she will periodically feel (palpate) your abdomen, to check how far down into the pelvis your baby's head has moved. She will also perform regular vaginal examinations to check the dilation of the cervix; note how often your contractions occur and how strong they are; take your blood pressure, temperature and pulse; and make notes about any pain relief that you have rquested and been given.

All of the information gathered by your midwife is noted on a chart known as a 'partogram'. If a change of shift takes place during your labour, the new team will use the partogram and a detailed handover to come up to speed with what's happening with your labour.

The early phase

When they begin, contractions tend to be mild. You'll feel a tightening in the abdomen, much like period pains, with some lower back pain, although the experience does vary. Contractions slowly become stronger, more frequent and more regularly spaced during this phase. This eventually changes the shape of the cervix (a process known as 'effacement'), making it shallower and softer (see opposite), so that it can dilate (open wide) enough to allow the baby to pass through it.

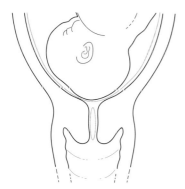

Before contractions begin, the cervix is closed, thin and around 2cm long.

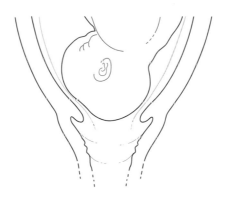

When the cervix is fully dilated to 10cm, the transition phase of labour begins, followed by the second stage, when you are ready to push.

At this point, you may be feeling tired and nauseous, so try to get as much rest as possible to conserve your energy for later. Try to manage the pain using deep breathing and relaxation techniques, massage and/or a TENS machine (see also box, opposite). Try a warm, soothing bath to ease the pain.

Waters breaking

Rupture of the membranes (or your waters breaking) usually occurs at some point in the first stage of labour, but it can happen at any time during labour. When the membranes containing your baby break, amniotic fluid leaks out. After this has taken place, the cervix dilates faster and the contractions speed up. In some circumstances, it may be necessary to rupture the membranes artificially. If this is the case with you, your obstetrician or midwife will explain why it is needed and first gain your consent.

The active phase

When your cervix has dilated to 3cm, your contractions are painful and regular, and the baby's head has moved downwards in the pelvis, you are officially in the active phase of labour, during which your contractions will become stronger, longer and more frequent. Typically, at the start of the active phase, you may have a contraction once every five minutes; by the end of the phase, they may occur once every two minutes or so, with a very short break in between them. During this phase the baby's head and shoulders slowly move further down in the pelvis.

Managing pain in the first stage

Maintaining your mental strength and focus during the first stage of labour can make all the difference between moving relatively gracefully through giving birth and becoming a wreck. Imagine that you are climbing a set of stairs and that each contraction is one step. With each step, you are getting closer to your goal of delivering your baby safely. Stay focused on each step alone until the contraction ends. Rest and relax as much as possible before the next step (contraction). Don't think about how many steps there are between you and your destination, or you could become disheartened. In any case, no one can know how far there is to go and you may be much closer than you think! Stay well hydrated with sips of water, and keep your energy levels topped up with regular snacks. Shift position from time to time, to remain comfortable, and try to keep your mind focused on something soothing and calming between your contractions. If you feel you can't cope with the pain, and that pain relief would help you to maintain your mental composure, ask for it, or more of it!

Try to remain upright, which will help your baby descend into the birth canal and into the best position for birth. If you can manage it, try walking around. The following positions can be comfortable:

✦ kneeling down, leaning forwards on a birthing ball, your birth partner or some pillows
✦ sitting, leaning forwards, being supported by your birth partner
✦ standing, leaning against a wall
✦ sitting on a birthing ball and rotating your hips
✦ kneeling down on all fours.

The transition phase

This is the final phase of the first stage of labour, but some women's bodies skip it. You move into this phase when you are 9–10cm dilated. It can last from a few minutes to an hour, during which your contractions are very frequent. By this time, you may have been in labour for a long time and may feel tired, cold, shivery and nauseous, and you may even vomit. It's easy to lose heart at this stage, so try to remember that you are very close to the end now. Your birth partner or partners should do all that they can to keep your spirits up, help you maintain your mental composure and support you through this particularly difficult phase.

Once you are 10cm dilated you are in the second stage of labour and your baby's head has descended low enough within the pelvis to be level with its narrowest point (at the level of the ischial spines). It is likely that you will feel the urge to push, and you will move into the second stage of labour (see opposite).

The Second Stage of Labour

This stage begins when your cervix is 10cm dilated. You may feel an intense urge to push. It won't be long now until you meet your baby.

Action time!

For a first labour, this stage usually takes longer than in subsequent labours and typically lasts for one to two hours, which reduces to less than an hour on average in subsequent labours. How long the second stage takes also depends on how effective your pushing is, how far down into the birth canal your baby has descended by the time you are fully dilated, how strong your contractions are, whether you can feel them (you may have had an epidural), how big the baby's head is, and the position of the baby (see page 102–3).

You may want to change the position you take a few times, or you might find a comfortable position for all of this stage. Try to remain as upright as possible during the second stage, so that gravity can do some of the work for you. Some women kneel on all fours with the hips lower than the shoulders; others prefer to sit on a birthing stool or on the edge of a bed. Squatting is a good position for birth, but it is difficult to remain squatting for a long time.

The pushing stage

Pushing happens mostly involuntarily if little or no pain relief has been used. It usually happens with each contraction after you are 10cm dilated. If the 'urge' to push has not yet happened, passive descent (which is when you allow the contractions to take their course while you wait for the urge to push) allows the baby to move lower into the pelvis, which is when the urge to push may come on. If not, a few practice pushes may kick-start the reflex. If you are using an epidural, you won't be able to feel the contractions or the urge to push, so your midwife will guide you through them. Listen very carefully to what your midwife tells you to do – she will explain how to breathe and when to push in order to make the most of each contraction.

Episiotomy

An episiotomy is a small cut made to the perineum. Episiotomies are performed to help a forceps delivery along, to speed up a delivery if necessary, if you are finding it hard to deliver the shoulders, if your baby is in the breech position, or if you've previously had a third-degree tear.

Some women need no help in pushing their babies out and use their instinct with the power of their contractions. Others needs some guidance, in which case the midwife will tell you to push down 'into your bottom'. Don't be embarrassed by this. A lot of women waste energy pushing into their abdomen. Instead, when the midwife tells you to push, take a deep breath, then close up the throat and push into your bottom as if trying very hard to pass a stool. During each contraction, you will have roughly three gos at this breathe-and-strong-pushing, which is better than holding your breath for the entire contraction (which could make you feel light-headed).

If you work with the midwife in this way, allowing her to guide you, you will be pushing the baby further down the birth canal with each contraction. It helps to imagine your baby moving down the birth canal as you work at it. As the baby gets closer to the vaginal opening, you might feel pain in your rectum and down your legs, and your anus may bulge outwards. This is because the baby's head is now putting pressure on the area. You might also pass a stool, as the baby's head pushes out any stools left in the bowel on its way out. Again, don't be embarrassed. You'd be surprised at how often this happens, and the midwives and obstetricians are all very used to it and see it as par for the course.

The midwife may examine you frequently during this stage to check your baby's position and your progress, although it is not always necessary because midwives are skilled at recognising the many external signs of progress. If, after you have been pushing for 90 minutes, delivery doesn't seem to be approaching, your midwife and the obstetrician may well discuss intervention measures, such as using forceps or a ventouse, or in certain cases having a Caesarean section.

Emerging baby

If all is progressing well, then the baby's hair will, in due course, become visible at the vaginal opening (although it will slide back in again at the end of each contraction).

Next, the head will 'crown' – this is when it has fully arrived at the opening and is soon to emerge, usually within a couple of contractions. Many women feel a stinging or burning sensation on the perineum at this point. Listen very carefully to what the midwife tells you to do during this crucial phase. She will guide you through when to push and exactly when and how to breathe, and her guidance will allow

Vaginal tearing

Many women sustain a vaginal tear, especially during very fast labours.

First-degree tears do not usually require stitches and tend to heal quickly and well. Second-degree tears are deeper tears that require stitching because the tear affects the layer of muscle of the perineum.

When it's time for you to be stitched up (usually within an hour of delivery, once the placenta has been delivered), you'll be asked to move to the end of the bed and put your legs onto leg rests, to enable the midwife or obstetrician to see clearly. If necessary, you'll be given another anaesthetic injection.

Third-degree tears are basically second-degree tears that involve the muscle of the anal sphincter.

In fourth-degree tears, not just the anus but also the skin or mucus lining of the rectum (just inside the anus) is torn.

Third- and fourth-degree tears are rare and need the attention of a senior doctor, who will stitch up the area with great skill, in order to avoid long-term problems such as faecal or flatulence incontinance. This is carried out in theatre, and if you need this type of repair you are given a spinal anaesthetic.

the head to emerge slowly, allowing the vaginal tissues and opening to stretch with the least risk or minimum amount of tearing. The midwife will guide you through the process of the baby's head emerging.

Once the head is out, the midwife will ensure that the umbilical cord is not coiled around the baby's neck, and will take it away from the neck if it is. She will guide you through the process as the baby's first shoulder, then the next one emerge during your next couple of contractions. The rest of your baby's body will come out soon afterwards.

Immediately after the birth

If your baby is healthy, she will take her first breath as soon as she emerges, and she will cry out. The midwife will put your baby on your chest straight away so you have skin-to-skin contact with her, covering her with a blanket to keep her warm. Soon after the birth, the midwife will clean her up and the umbilical cord will be cut (see page 114).

The midwife or a paediatrician (a doctor specialising in the health of babies and children) will examine your baby's heart rate, respiratory effort, reflexes, tone and colour at 1 minute, 5 minutes and 10 minutes of age, usually without needing to remove her from your arms, to produce your baby's Apgar score. This scoring system is used to

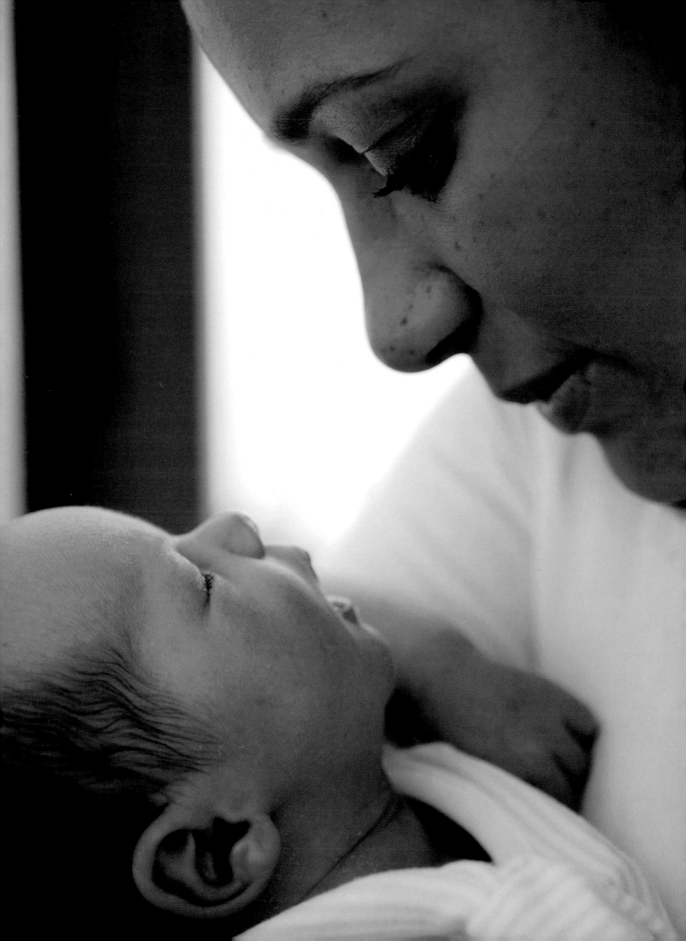

assess the condition of babies at birth. If your baby's score is 7 or higher, it means her condition is good; a result of 4–6 indicates she needs help to breathe; a result of 3 or less means that emergency attention may be required. The test is repeated because, in some cases, the score changes within minutes, so the midwife is alerted to these changes. Don't worry if the results are not high – this does not mean that there is definitely something wrong. In the vast majority of cases, a low score at 1 minute will improve at 5 minutes. Apgar scoring is simply a way of assessing the help a baby requires in the minutes after birth. Your healthcare providers will continue to monitor your baby over the next few hours.

If the midwife has been concerned about your baby's heart rate during the birth, she may ask for blood samples from the umbilical cord straight after the delivery, to check your baby's oxygen supply during the birth has been normal. The results of these tests are available in a few minutes and will help your healthcare providers decide whether or not your baby should be transferred to the neonatal unit for monitoring.

If your baby is doing well, she'll be weighed and checked for physical abnormalities. The midwife will attach a hospital identity bracelet to each of her ankles showing your name, the baby's hospital number, and a date and time of birth. She will ask whether you know about the vitamin K injection given to newborn babies and discuss its use. If you give your consent, she will administer it to your baby soon after birth.

How you feel

Everyone's experience of labour is unique, and there is no right or wrong way to feel at this moment. You're likely to feel completely exhausted, especially if the labour has been long, or you may feel invigorated by the amazing feat your body has performed. You may have the shakes and feel shivery. Many women have a strong physical response to labour.

You may feel euphoric, full of joy, delighted finally to see your baby. You may feel out of it, bemused and confused, as if you can't quite believe it's all really over. Many women feel both delighted and terrified at the same time! It's a sobering thought, especially if it's your first baby, that you are responsible for this new person who is entirely dependent on you. This can create feelings of protectiveness and love as the mothering instinct kicks in. But some women don't feel very interested in the baby because they are exhausted. Don't worry if you feel this way. As long as your baby is on your chest, skin to skin, she'll feel happy. Allow yourself to rest – there's plenty of time for you to get to know your baby.

The Third Stage of Labour

The third stage begins once the baby is born. First, the umbilical cord is cut, after which you will deliver the placenta. Delivering the placenta is the unglamorous bit that you certainly won't recognise from the movies!

Cutting the umbilical cord

Your midwife will wait for a couple of minutes before cutting the umbilical cord, which is good for the baby, then she will position two clamps near one another in the middle section of the cord. Either she or your partner (if he wants to cut the cord) will then cut it between the clamps. The stump will eventually dry out and fall off, revealing your baby's belly button. The midwife will tell you how to care for, it to ensure that it doesn't become infected.

Delivering the placenta

There are two approaches to delivering the placenta. The most common is called 'active management of the third stage'. The other is known as 'traditional management of the third stage'.

Active management

The advantage of active management of the third stage is that it makes the third stage happen quickly, slightly reducing the risk of heavy bleeding (haemorrhaging). It can, however, cause headaches and nausea.

If you opt for active management of the third stage (which you would do in consultation with your midwife during an antenatal check up), you will receive an injection in your thigh during the second stage of labour of either a drug called Syntometrine or one called Syntocinon, once the baby's head and one shoulder have been delivered. This makes your contractions longer and the womb shrink in size rapidly, which causes the placenta to detach quickly and come out through the cervix, emerging from the vaginal opening. The midwife will monitor all of this. When there are signs that the placenta has separated from the wall of the womb the midwife will place one hand on your abdomen and gently pull on the umbilical cord, to encourage the placenta to come out.

Retained placenta

In a small minority of cases (approximately 1 per cent), the placenta remains inside the womb. If this is the case at an hour after delivering the baby, the obstetrician in charge will order either a general or regional anaesthetic, and will then manually remove the placenta. This procedure will take place in an operating theatre.

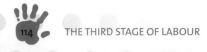

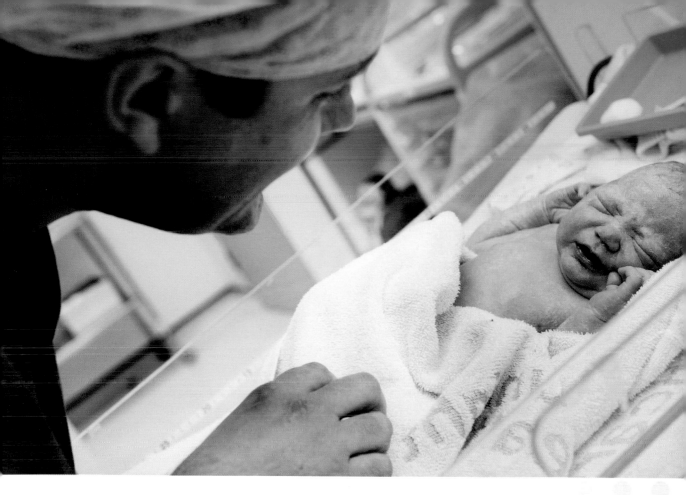

Traditional management

This natural approach to delivering the placenta uses no drugs to speed up the process, but there is a small but greater risk of severe bleeding (haemorrhaging). It can take up to an hour for the placenta to come away from the wall of the womb, but breastfeeding can help, as it releases a hormone that causes the womb to contract. The midwife will establish that the placenta is no longer attached – you'll experience some bleeding and may feel the urge to push, indicating that the placenta is free and ready to come out. The process takes roughly 20 minutes on average.

What happens next?

Once the placenta is delivered, the midwife will check that you are not bleeding, and that it is all there. It's likely to have emerged in one piece, but if it has broken up she will piece it together, to ensure that none of it has been left behind. If you need stitches due to tearing or an episiotomy (see boxes on pages 110–11), these will be done now, then you will have a wash. Some women can breastfeed while being stiFinally, you, your partner and your baby will be left alone to get to know each other.

Pain Relief in Labour

When it comes to pain relief during labour, you have a variety of options to choose from, from medical drugs to complementary therapies. Learn about your options in advance, so that you can prepare for using them, if necessary, and what to expect, so that you can make the right decisions for yourself on the day.

Making informed choices

Most women approach childbirth with some sort of plan in place for how they will tackle the pain involved using one or more forms of pain relief. This is a good idea because pain causes tension at best and can be utterly exhausting and traumatising at worst.

Some medical drugs remove the pain altogether, while non-medical pain-relief options help you to manage the pain so that you can tolerate it better. Read about the different options, so that you are ready for your labour and birth – and for making last-minute decisions about pain relief on the day. The choice is yours, and you can change your mind at the last minute, too (so keep your options open). Don't let anyone talk you into a drug-free birth if you feel you would rather have pain relief (or vice versa, if it's important for you to try to give birth without pain relief), or insist you use a particular type of pain relief if you don't like the sound of it.

Analgesia

Gas and air

Entonox, often referred to as 'gas and air', is the most common form of pain relief used in labour, with more than 80 per cent of women relying on it, especially during early labour. It doesn't completely block out the pain, but it can lessen it. Many women find it very helpful in dealing with the pain, although the effects of it are very short-lived, so you have to keep taking it. It comes in a cylinder, or is piped through the wall, with a mouthpiece attached by a tube. You take a deep inhalation at the start of the contraction and continue to do throughout and, by the time the contraction peaks, that 'hit' of gas and air will have kicked in enough to reduce the pain. It is perfectly safe to use and does not affect your baby. Some women feel light-headed and nauseous in response to it, or find it

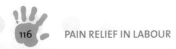

doesn't help with the pain at all. It does help many women, however, and concentrating on your breathing can help to keep you calm. You can have gas and air at a home birth, at a birthing centre or at the hospital.

Pethidine

This drug is a good choice for women who want to avoid using regional anaesthetic and who are having a normal, complication-free delivery. It is used by a third of labouring women, and is given as an injection to the thigh. It takes 15–20 minutes to kick in, and lasts for up to 4 hours. A second dose is available for use if your labour lasts longer than that. It's a powerful relaxant, and while it does not remove the pain, most people who have it relax better between contractions and care a lot less about them when they come! Midwives are able to prescribe and administer pethidine so this means you can have it at home, at a birthing centre or at the hospital. You might be offered meptazinol or diamorphine instead, but they all have the same effect and do not harm either you or your baby. Pethidine does cross the placenta and can result in a baby needing stimulation to breathe when born. Usually, this is not the case. If help is needed, it will be only minimally and an antidote to pethidine is readily available. Side effects include nausea and vomiting, and drowsiness, and many women say they feel a bit dazed.

Regional analgesia

Epidural anaesthetic

An epidural is used by 40 per cent of first-time mothers. It is usually given at the mother's request or in long, stalled labours. It is used for Caesarean sections and for women who are obese, which makes it difficult to administer regional anaesthetic in an emergency. Research shows that epidurals are safe, and it is very rare to be injured by one.

The anaesthetist will tell you exactly how to sit or lie, then will give you a local anaesthetic injection into your lower back before inserting the epidural needle, which contains a tiny tube called the 'epidural catheter'. This remains in place once the needle is removed, so that your dose can be topped up. It takes about 20 minutes to prepare the anesthesia and, once you've had it, it takes roughly half an hour to kick in. Your tummy area will feel completely numb. Your legs may also feel numb, and you may not be able to tell when you need to pee, so a urinary catheter will be used to take care of your bladder during this important time. You won't be aware of your contractions or any urge to push, but the midwife will tell you when and what to do. You will be able to push, despite not being able to feel in the area. Your pushing might not be as strong as it would without the epidural, but it should be strong enough for you to be able to deliver your baby. The chances of needing an assisted delivery (see pages 122–3) are higher when having an epidural, due to the lack of urge to push and sometimes ineffective pushing. To combat this, when the mother is 10cm dilated, it is common practice to get her to wait for one hour before starting the active pushing, which allows her contractions do more work for her and bring the baby a little closer, making it easier to push out the baby.

Side effects are experienced by very few women. Some get a headache after the birth, while others may feel tingling or have numbness in a leg. All symptoms disappear within a few days or, in even rarer cases, a few weeks.

Pudendal block
Pudendal blocks reduce the amount of pain felt in the vagina and perineum, and so they tend to be used for assisted deliveries (see pages 122–3), but they are not useful for labouring women because they don't remove the pain of contractions. The anaesthetic is injected inside the vagina, near the cervix, and the pain relief kicks in after 5–10 minutes.

Spinal block
These are used mostly for Caesarean sections and emergency interventions, as they take effect immediately. The effects don't last for more than 1–2 hours, the drug can be administered only once, and you are numb from mid-chest to your feet and unable to move, which means that they are not useful as pain relief during labour. Spinal blocks are used in theatre and for assisted deliveries in the event of a drawn-out pushing stage. They are also used if a placenta must be removed by hand and when repairing third or fourth-degree tears.

General anaesthetic
Very few women having a Caesarean section would prefer to be asleep during the procedure, although if that's the case a general anaesthetic can be discussed with your healthcare providers. Mostly, a 'general' is given only in extreme emergencies, if there has been massive bleeding or if your blood does not clot efficiently. A surgical delivery with the mother under general anaesthetic usually lasts for three-quarters of an hour to an hour. You will regain consciousness very soon after the surgery, at which point you will be moved to a recovery room and monitored until the nurses are satisfied with your progress. After this, you will be moved to the postnatal ward. Your baby will be with you the entire time.

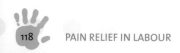

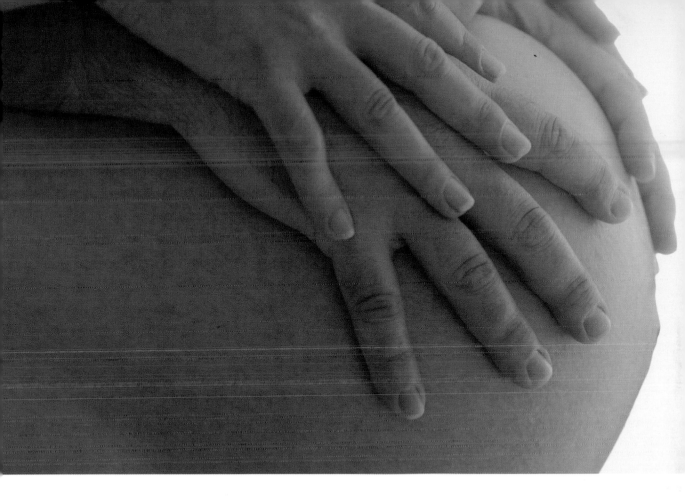

Non-medical pain relief

Many women use complementary therapies and natural methods to help with labour pains. Relaxing and focusing on something other than your pain can help you cope with contractions, so that you're less likely to tense up and release stress hormones that make the pain seem more intense. Some forms of non-medical pain relief are particularly popular with pregnant and labouring women. If you like the idea of any of the below, research so that you can assess them. You'll need a qualified practitioner for hypnotherapy, acupuncture and reflexology, and do check with the hospital or birthing centre (if you're not having a home birth) that they are allowed to attend the birth. Popular therapies include:

✦ breathing exercises
✦ massage
✦ reflexology
✦ aromatherapy
✦ homeopathy/herbalism
✦ acupuncture
✦ hypnobirthing
✦ TENS machine (see page 106).

Induced Labour

In some instances, labour has to be artificially started, which your midwife or obstetrician will talk you through at your 40-week appointment. They will be keen to see your baby born before 42 weeks and will book you for an induction when you reach 40 weeks plus 12 days.

Membrane sweep

If at 40 or 41 weeks you have not gone into labour, you will be offered a membrane sweep. The midwife runs a finger around the cervix, which can cause the membranes to separate from the cervix and the cervix to ripen, ready for birth. This may be enough to start your contractions, which means you avoid having more invasive forms of induction (see below).

Induction: reasons and risks

Roughly 25 per cent of labours are induced, mostly because a baby is overdue. Your obstetrician will suggest induction if concerned about your baby's or your health, and feels an earlier delivery would be best, or if your labour has not begun 24 hours after your waters broke. There are a few risks that come with induction. There is a slightly higher risk of needing an assisted delivery or a Caesarean section, along with hyperstimulation of the womb, and the first stage of labour is likely to be longer.

Induction methods

Three methods are used to induce labour. Your healthcare providers will tell you which is most suitable for your circumstances.

Prostaglandin

The body produces this hormone to stimulate contractions. A synthetic version is made in the form of a gel, pessary or tablet, which is inserted into the vagina, causing the cervix to ripen and contractions to begin.

Artificial rupture of the membranes (ARM)

If there is a medical reason for not giving you prostaglandins, your obstetrician may suggest ARM, in which he or she will insert a long, hooked needle into the vagina and pierce the membranes (the 'bag'

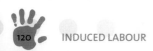

containing your baby and the amniotic fluid). You need to be at least 1–2cm dilated, if this is your first labour, for this procedure (in subsequent labours, the cervix is already a little open due to previous childbirth). Breaking the membranes in this way can bring on contractions. This procedure may feel uncomfortable.

Syntocinon

This is a synthetic version of the hormone oxytocin, which is made by the body to stimulate contractions. It is given as a drip into the arm or hand. The dosage begins at a low level, but is adjusted in response to how well the body responds to it. The disadvantage is that Syntocinon brings on strong contractions quickly, so the body has no opportunity to adapt to increasingly stronger contractions over time. As a result, many women opt for an epidural when they are induced using Syntocinon.

Going in for an induction

Once admitted, your temperature and blood pressure are taken. The midwife examines you internally, to check the ripeness of your cervix, and feels your abdomen to see if the baby's head is engaged (see page 103).

You will then be given a prostaglandin pessary, tablet or gel, which will be inserted into your vagina. After this, you will simply wait for your contractions to start, so take a good book, magazines, some music or another way of passing the time to the hospital with you. It's unlikely that anything will happen for a while – in a first labour, you are unlikely to deliver for at least 36 hours after first insertion. If all goes well and your body responds to the prostaglandin, your contractions will begin and your waters will break, and you will be moved to a delivery room once your labour is established.

If your body does not respond to prostaglandin, and you took a 6-hour version, your baby's heartbeat will be checked, you will be asked to walk around, (which can sometimes kick-start contractions), then you will be assessed again 6 hours later. You may then repeat the entire procedure two more times. After that, if your body doesn't respond to prostaglandin, your obstetrician may suggest you wait for a day to see what happens, you progress to the Syntocinon method of induction, or you have a Caesarean section.

If you took the 24-hour option, your baby's heartbeat will be monitored and you will be asked to wait for up to 24 hours for your contractions to begin. If there are still no contractions, the obstetrician will suggest a Caesarean section.

Augmented labour

Sometimes, in labours in which contractions have started by themselves, both the contractions and the dilation of the cervix slow down. In order to make further progress, the obstetrician might suggest ARM (if the waters haven't yet broken) or Syntocinon in a low dose, to help get the contractions going again.

Assisted Deliveries

There are two methods of assisted delivery: the use of ventouse (suction cup) and forceps. If your labour is not progressing as it should, your obstetrician may recommend one of these methods.

Reasons for an assisted delivery

Ventouse or forceps are used in roughly 15 per cent of births, two-thirds of which use ventouse and one-third forceps. The obstetrician may suggest assistance if the baby's position is transverse or posterior (see page 102), the baby shows signs of distress or 'fetal compromise' (his heartbeat is abnormally high or low, meaning his oxygen supply may be compromised), if there is meconium (see page 105) in the amniotic fluid, if you are unable to push enough to get the baby out due to an epidural, or if the baby is not moving down in the birth canal when the cervix is fully dilated. Pain relief is provided for the procedure (if you haven't had some), and your legs are suspended in leg rests so that the midwife or obstetrician can see clearly.

Ventouse

For this method, the cervix must be fully dilated, and the baby's head must be a good way down the birth canal. A plastic or metal cup is fitted to the top of the baby's head. The cup has a long tube attached that's in turn attached to a suction device that creates a vacuum in the cup, attaching it to the baby's head within two minutes. There is a handle fitted to the cup so it can be gently pulled by the midwife or obstetrician to guide out the baby. The mother needs to push out the baby, but the ventouse helps her to deliver. The cup is removed once the head crowns (see page 110) and the mother then continues to push out the baby.

Once the baby is born, a 'chignon' (area of swelling at the site of the cup) is visible, which reduces after some days. In rare cases, there is bruising on the site that takes two or three weeks to heal. In even rarer cases, the bruising is extreme and causes jaundice, or there is intercranial bleeding.

A ventouse-assisted delivery carries less risk of perineal damage. The method can help to encourage a baby to turn from a tricky position into the ideal occipito-anterior position (see page 102–3).

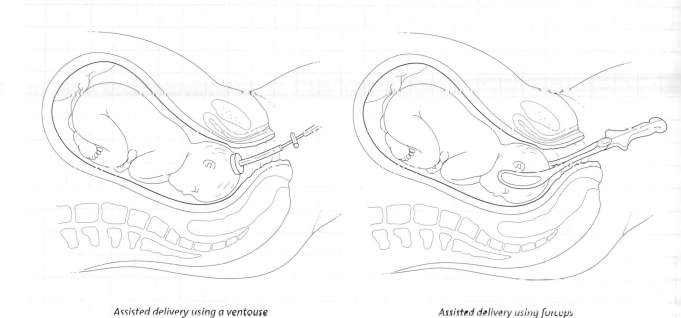

Assisted delivery using a ventouse

Assisted delivery using forceps

Forceps

Forceps will be suggested if delivery needs to be aided rapidly (ventouse takes a couple of minutes to set up), if the mother is unable to push, if the baby is tired or distressed, and in other cases. There are three types – low, lift-out forceps, straight traction forceps and rotational forceps. Each type is inserted one blade at a time into the vagina and into position with one against each side of the head. The obstetrician gently pulls as you push out the baby. The vaginal opening must enlarged by episiotomy (see page 110) to allow both forceps and baby's head to fit through and avoid tearing.

If the baby's head is almost delivered but the mother needs a little help or the baby seems distressed or tired, a midwife might use low, lift-out forceps to assist the delivery. If the head is engaged and has moved some way down the birth canal, straight traction forceps can be used to deliver the baby by pulling gently on the forceps during contractions. Usually, three or four strong contractions is all it takes to deliver the head in this way. After the birth, the baby's head may seem bruised at the sides, where the forceps were applied, but this subsides within a few days.

With forceps, the baby's head rotate as it navigates the birth canal (because it is not held in position) with suction cup attached, and the vaginal opening doesn't necessarily require widening with an episiotomy.

Breech Birth

Delivering a breech baby is a tricky affair and, consequently, roughly 90 per cent of babies in breech presentation are born by Caesarean section. However, it is not an impossible task.

Vaginal or Caesarean delivery?

The results of numerous studies show that delivering a breech baby by Caesarean section is safer than delivering vaginally. There are a number of risks associated with delivering a breech baby vaginally. Fetal compromise (see page 122) is more likely, as breech deliveries generally take longer than normal ones, and there is a greater chance of a prolapsed umbilical cord (see page 97), which can be dangerous to the baby. Also, the baby's body can pass through the cervix when it is not yet 10cm dilated, so the head can get stuck. This necessitates a dangerous emergency procedure that is best avoided by performing a Caesarean section earlier on in proceedings. Roughly 4 per cent of babies are in a breech position at 36–37 weeks. If yours is breech, your midwife will talk you through your delivery options.

Breech presentation

There are three breech positions. In the frank breech, the baby's bottom 'presents' (is closest to the cervix and will be the first part to be delivered), and the baby's legs are stretched out and extended upwards. Babies in this breech presentation are most successfully delivered vaginally. In a flexed or complete breech, the bottom is, again, presenting, but the knees are bent in front of the baby and the feet are downwards. In a footling breech the legs are low in front of the body and a foot is presenting, making a vaginal delivery hard. Your obstetrician may suggest a Caesarean section.

External cephalic version (ECV)

If your baby is in a breech presentation, an ECV may be done at 37 weeks. The baby is encouraged to turn to a head-down position by pressure applied to the mother's abdomen. The procedure can be uncomfortable, and you may be given a drug to relax the womb muscle. There is a 50 per cent success rate with ECV in first pregnancies, rising to 60–70 per cent in

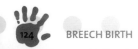

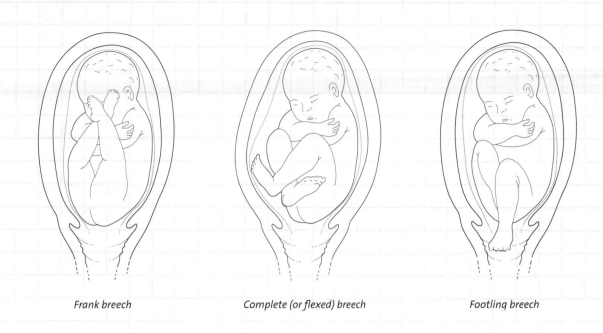

| Frank breech | Complete (or flexed) breech | Footling breech |

subsequent pregnancies. There are some circumstances in which it is unadvisable, so you may not be offered one. If this is the case, if it doesn't work or if you would rather not have the procedure, you might book a Caesarean section or deliver the baby vaginally. Your obstetrician will talk you through your options and explain the pros and cons of each.

Delivery of a breech baby

If you try to deliver a breech baby vaginally, it will be considered a 'trial', with the operating theatre readily available for an emergency Caesarean section. You'll be closely observed, and supervised by a senior obstetrician and midwife throughout. You'll be advised to have an epidural because the procedures used in the final stages of delivery can be painful and because you will then be ready for surgery if the need arises.

If you get to the pushing stage, the midwife or obstetrician may ask you to rest on a bed with your feet in leg rests, so they have access. The bottom emerges first, followed by the legs, one at a time. The obstetrician, then begins to support the baby as the torso, arms and shoulders are delivered. Finally, the head is delivered. The obstetrician rests the baby on an arm and places the hand in front of the baby's face, with a finger on each side of the nose to support the face. The other hand is on the back of the baby's head, with a finger on the back of the head to guide it along the final stretch of the birth canal and out of the vaginal opening.

Caesarean Section

Between 25 and 30 per cent of births in the UK are achieved by Caesarean section. The figure rises to one-third in women over 35. As your chances of delivering by Caesarean are statistically high, it makes sense to learn what to expect.

Planned vs unplanned

If a Caesarean section is planned, it is called an 'elective' Caesarean. If it is unplanned, and happens because the need for it arose before or during a planned vaginal delivery, it is termed an emergency Caesarean. Roughly two-thirds of all Caesarean sections are 'emergency' Caesareans. The term 'emergency' is somewhat misleading, as it is rare that either mother or baby is in any urgent danger. In many cases, as long as the baby is born within half an hour, it is considered a safe delivery. In fact, obstetricians use a classification system to determine in each case how urgent the need for surgery is, and schedule surgeries according to it.

Elective Caesareans

There are several reasons for planning a Caesarean section.

If you have placenta praevia, in which the placenta's position obscures or blocks the cervix, your obstetrician will tell you that a Caesarean is the only safe way to deliver your baby.

If your baby is unwell and needs surgery soon after she is born, planning a Caesarean will allow your healthcare team to make the necessary arrangements to ensure the right staff are available for the baby.

In cases where the baby is in a breech or transverse position (see pages 124–5), the obstetrician may try to turn the baby. However, if that fails, and you don't want to try to deliver the baby vaginally, you can choose to have a Caesarean. About 90 per cent of breech presentations are delivered by Caesarean section.

If you have delivered by Caesarean section in the past and you don't want to try a vaginal delivery, you can book a Caesarean. But bear in mind that roughly three-quarters of women who have had a previous Caesarean go on to have successful vaginal deliveries.

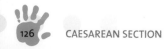

If your obstetrician or midwife suggests a Caesarean, they will discuss the reasons for the suggestion, and the pros and cons of surgery in your specific case. You may decide that having an elective Caesarean is the safest choice (or, indeed, the only choice) due to your circumstances, or you may decide with your healthcare providers that it is OK to try for a vaginal delivery, knowing that the operating theatre is not far away, should you need it.

If you want a Caesarean despite there being no medical reason why you should have one, you are within your rights to request one. Your healthcare team will explore your reasons with you and assess them.

Emergency Caesareans

Problems do come up during deliveries that make it necessary to deliver the baby sooner rather than later or, in some circumstances, as soon as possible. For example, umbilical cord prolapse might occur, putting the baby in grave danger, or if the baby's heart rate becomes abnormal and/or meconium is present (see page 105) and there may be fetal compromise (see page 122). In some cases, labour stops progressing well, perhaps because the cervix doesn't dilate enough or because contractions slow down in frequency and intensity. Heavy maternal bleeding could be caused by any of a few problems that require urgent attention. If the decision has been made to deliver a very premature baby for reasons such as severe pre-eclampsia, a Caesarean section is preferred because these tiny babies do not tolerate labour well.

Most usually, if the need for an emergency Caesarean occurs, it takes up to an hour before your baby or you are at risk. Problems sometimes arise soon before labour is due to begin that make it clear that you will need to have a Caesarean. You may know that a Caesarean may be on the cards as you begin what your healthcare team labels a slightly risky labour, only to find that you do need a Caesarean in the end. All of these instances would be considered emergency Caesareans, as the procedure was not planned and booked in advance.

The operating theatre

The operation takes place in an operating theatre, on an operating table. There are bright lights so that the team can clearly see what is going on. Various machines, medicines and trolleys are in the room. At the head-end of the bed will be the anaesthetist's equipment. The team will erect a fabric screen between you and the site of the surgery. Your birth partner will be allowed into the theatre with you, but will need to wear scrubs, as will all the medical staff present.

The medical team

Expect to see a number of people in the theatre during your surgery. The obstetrician leads the team and performs the surgery, and an assistant obstetrician helps the obstetrician during the operation. The anaesthetist administers the anaesthetic, with an assistant anaesthetist or an operating department assistant to help. There are theatre nurses present, to check the equipment and pass instruments to the obstetrician upon request. The midwife will be there to help once your baby has been delivered, and a paediatrician wil be there to check the baby is fine and carry out the Apgar scoring (see page 111–13).

The procedure

The delivery itself takes no more than five minutes to perform, but the entire procedure will take roughly an hour. The anaesthetic takes a little time to prepare, and the staff spend some time preparing your for surgery. Plus after the surgery, the stitching up of your womb, the muscle layers of your abdomen, and your skin takes up more time.

The midwives will ask you to put on a hospital gown and surgical stockings before you get to theatre, and also ask you to remove jewellery, make-up and nail varnish. In theatre, you will be asked to lie down on an operating table and will have a clip monitor attached to a finger, to check your oxygen levels throughout the surgery. Your blood pressure will also be monitored every minute. Next, while the other members of staff prepare for the surgery, the anaesthetist will prepare and administer the anaesthetic.

The anaesthetic

In most cases, the mother is awake during the surgery. The anaesthetist will assess your case and establish which is the best form of anaesthetic in your case. It might be an epidural, a CSE (a combined spinal epidural for surgeries in which complications are anticipated, as it may outlast a spinal block, see page 118). He or she will then set up the chosen form of anaesthetic, and a saline drip will also be set up and inserted into your arm.

Next, the anaesthetist will run some tests to make sure that you can't feel anything at the operation site. Once the team is completely sure the aneasthetic is working effectively, they will begin to prepare you for the operation.

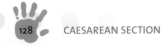

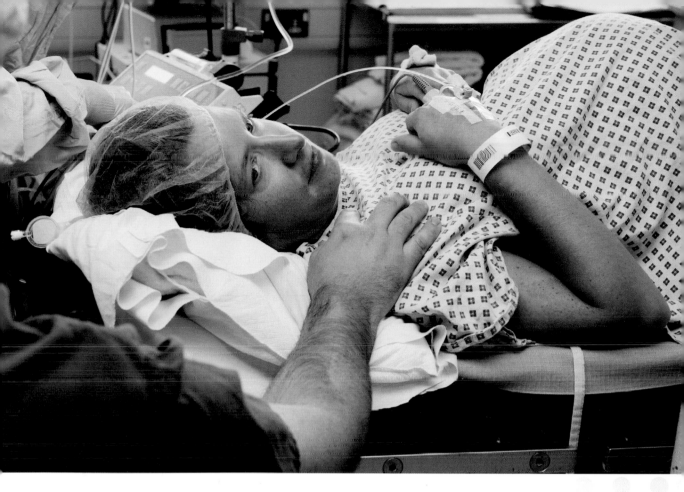

Prepping the mother

A catheter will be inserted into your urethra, so that your bladder can drain during the surgery and for the 12 or so hours afterwards, when it will be difficult to get up and walk to the toilet. (It will be taken out only when you are sure that you can manage to walk to the loo alone.)

Someone in the medical team will clip your pubic hair in the area of the planned incision, then give your abdominal area a wash with antiseptic solution. Your legs will be covered in sterile sheeting, as will the upper part of your abdomen, so that only the operation site is visible to the team. The screen between you and the operation site will then be erected. Ask the team to lower it if you would like to see your baby emerging.

The birth

The team is now ready for the surgery. First, the obstetrician makes the cut, which will be right at the base of your abdomen, just above the pubic bone. It will be roughly 15cm long. There are a few layers to cut through – first the skin, then fat and muscle tissue, then into the womb itself. If your waters haven't yet broken, the obstetrician will break the membranes.

The rise in Caesareans

The amount of babies born by Caesarean section has been steadily rising because it's a much safer procedure than it was, so obstetricians won't hesitate to use it if necessary. Also, improvement in the technologies of diagnostic equipment, such as ultrasound scanning make it easier to detect problems with the baby while she is in the womb. Caesarean sections planned in order to arrange the baby's medical care post-birth take place more frequently. There are also social reasons for the increase in the rate of Caesareans. More women over 35 are having babies – and first babies – than in the past, and complications are statistically more likely to arise during pregnancy and labour in women of this age group. Also, because there is more obesity in recent years, there are more obese pregnant women, for whom complications are more likely to arise during labour and, therefore, are more likely to lead to a Caesarean.

Everyone has an opinion on whether Caesarean section is good or bad. Some people believe Caesareans are frequently given when there is a good chance for a mother to have delivered her baby vaginally. Others feel that there is no good reason to not use the procedure when available, especially if there is a risk to the baby. The most important thing about pregnancy and childbirth is the delivery of a healthy baby.

Next, the obstetrician will establish the exact position of your baby within the womb, to decide how best to take him out. If your baby is in a head-down position, the obstetrician will carefully lift it out of your pelvis through the incision. If another part of your baby's body was the presenting part (see page 124–5), it's likely the obstetrician will lift this out first because it is closest to the incision. If your baby's position makes it difficult to squeeze him through the incision site, the obstetrician may use forceps while the assistant obstetrician applies pressure on the abdomen, to help shift your baby into a more favourable position. While all of this is going on, you won't feel any pain at all, or be able to feel what exactly is going on, but you will feel a strange tugging sensation in your abdominal area.

As soon as the baby is delivered, the cord will be clamped and cut (see page 114) and the baby will be taken to the resuscitaire not far from you to be assessed by the paediatrician, then wrapped and given to you so you can marvel at him without interruption for a little while as the team performs the next stage of the procedure.

If your baby urgently needs the support of a neonatal unit, he will be taken there immediately after birth and placed in an incubator, so that his medical care can continue. This separation can be difficult for you, but if your baby needs the help you will feel grateful that it is there for him.

Finishing off

The placenta is delivered next. You will receive an intravenous injection of carbetocin or Syntocinon as per an actively managed third stage in a vaginal delivery (see page 114). The placenta and membranes will be removed from the womb through the incision, then the obstetrician will check the womb to ensure that it is empty, while the midwife checks the placenta to make sure it is intact or complete (see page 115).

Once the team is satisfied that the womb is empty, the process of stitching you up, layer by layer will begin. You and the baby will then be moved to the recovery area.

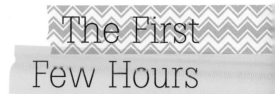

The First Few Hours

It's now time for you to get to know your baby, and the first few hours after the birth might be spent gazing at her in wonder! Your medical team, on the other hand, will want to know that both of you are doing well and are on the right track.

Time to recuperate

No doubt you are excited to be finally meeting your baby, but bear in mind that both of you need rest in order to recover from the birth. Babies tend to be sleepy for the first day or so, so try to sleep whenever your baby does, to give your body a chance to recuperate.

If you've had a home birth, all the same checks as done at the hospital after a birth will be done for you and your baby at home (see page 115). The midwives will clear up any birth-related mess and remove it from your home, along with the placenta, unless you specifically request them not to. The midwife will stay at your home for roughly two hours to make sure you and the baby are doing well before she leaves.

Your baby's appearance

A baby that has been delivered vaginally can look a little alarming to a first-time parent after the birth. The skin is wrinkly, perhaps patchy in colouration, the eyes are swollen and puffy, and there may be bruises where forceps or a ventouse suction cup was used (see page 122–3). Unless the midwife has cleaned up your baby before handing her to you, her skin will have a covering of vernix caseosa (see page 56), which is a white and greasy substance. She may also have a light covering of lanugo (see page 62). If she does, this soft, fine hair will come off over the next couple of weeks. If your baby is Caucasion, her eye colour at birth will be deep blue. If she is African or Asian, her eyes will be dark grey or brown. They will take on their genetic colour over the next few weeks.

If you delivered your baby vaginally then, most noticeably, your baby's head will be cone-shaped or weirdly long-looking! The head took on this shape as the bones at the top of the skull overlapped during birth, and will return to its usual shape within a few days.

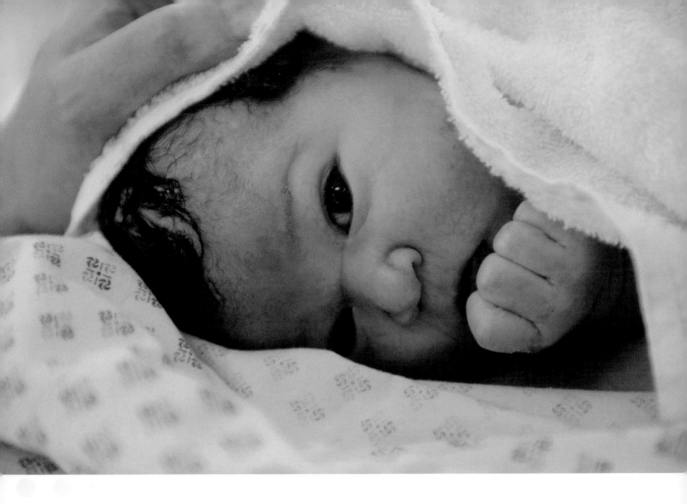

The genitals (in both boys and girls) are likely to be swollen because the baby received plenty of pregnancy hormones while in the mother's body. The breasts may leak some milk, and baby girls might have some vaginal discharge. Don't worry – this is normal. If a boy's testes are not yet descended, they will do so within a few weeks.

How you are feeling

You'll probably be feeling both utter elation and complete exhaustion after delivering your baby, especially if the labour was long. All you may want to do is sleep and gaze at her! Tell your would-be visitors to wait until tomorrow if you feel you want the rest and privacy. How you feel affects the baby, so focus on keeping yourself fighting fit.

You might feel hungry, especially if you didn't keep much food or water down during labour. You might have aches and pains in the abdominal region, known as afterpains. These are likely to continue for a few more days, especially when breastfeeding, as your reproductive organs slowly return to normal. If the pains are very strong, let the midwives know. They can give you painkillers to make you more comfortable.

Your pelvic-floor muscles have taken a battering during labour, and many women find that they suffer from incontinence of either the bladder or the bowel for a few days after the birth. Don't worry – this is normal, even after a Caesarean section, and the majority of women experience incontinence after birth. Remember that the sooner you start practising your pelvic-floor exercises again (see page 19), the quicker your bowel and bladder control will return to normal. The midwives will ask you to pass urine at least twice before you leave the hospital, to reassure themselves that your bladder is working fine after the birth. This is because a full bladder that you may not be able to empty can prevent the womb contracting and reducing in size, which is what stops the bleeding.

After a Caesarean section

About an hour after the surgery, you will begin to feel sensations in your legs. Your saline drip will be removed within the first four hours, and the catheter will be removed roughly 12 hours after surgery.

Once the anaesthetic has worn off, the midwives will give you painkillers to help you deal with the pain of the incision. These morphine-based painkillers are very strong, and you can request ibuprofen, paracetamol, diclofenac or naproxen after 24 hours. These are all fine to take if you are breastfeeding. Discuss the use of painkillers with a midwife before you leave the hospital, so that you can make sure you manage your pain effectively

If your skin feels very itchy, let your midwives know. This may be a reaction to the anaesthetic, for which they can give you medication to help you feel more comfortable.

In some hospitals your partner will be allowed to stay with you for the first night, which can be very helpful as you are unlikely to be back on your feet and able to go to the loo on your own. The midwives will want to see you up within 24 hours of the surgery, as this will reduce the risk of VTE (venous thromboembolism, which includes deep vein thrombosis and pulmonary embolism, which can be fatal).

It's never easy when you first start to move around after a Caesarean section, as your incision site will be sore. You'll quickly discover how difficult it is to perform very basic everyday tasks, let alone look after your baby, because you can't twist your body to either side, and even picking up your baby puts strain on the incision site. Make sure you ask for help. Don't be shy! If you sneeze, cough or laugh, hold on to your abdominal area to support it.

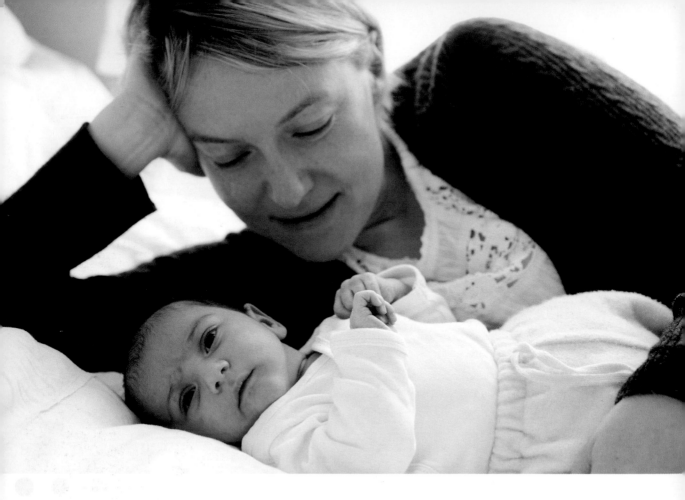

Lochia

Every woman bleeds heavily after giving birth (known as 'lochia'), which can last up to six weeks, gradually lessening in intensity. Women who have delivered vaginally tend to bleed more, as much of the blood, mucus and womb tissue in lochia is removed during a Caesarean section. Make sure that you are ready for this with a good supply of heavy-duty sanitary pads and some disposable knickers. From time to time you will feel a rush of blood from the vagina, or pass a clot. Neither of these is anything to worry about unless the bleeding continues to be heavy, the clots are large in size or the smell of the blood becomes offensive. These symptoms can be a sign of retained products such as a small piece of placenta or membrane, which will need monitoring and possibly removal.

Feeding your baby

If you intend to breastfeed your baby, the midwives or a breastfeeding specialist at the hospital can help you to learn how to do it. If you intend to bottle-feed your baby, these first few formula feeds will be provided by the hospital.

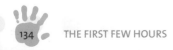

Breastfeeding

If you have chosen to breastfeed your baby, take your baby to your breast as soon as she is born if possible. If you are feeling unsure about what to do, ask the midwives, maternity support staff or a hospital lactation consultant for guidance. After that, offer your baby the breast regularly. Hopefully, she will learn how to suckle (or her sucking reflex will kick in quickly) and she will receive some nourishment from the colostrum your body produces for the first few days, before your milk comes in. Colostrum is high in many nutrients, giving your baby an immediate nutritional boost.

Time to leave the hospital

If you had a normal vaginal delivery, it's likely that you will leave the hospital within 24 hours. Most women who have had an assisted birth or a Caesarean section tend to stay for a day or two. The midwives and a paediatrician will assess you and the baby before you leave, to ensure that you are both well enough to go.

Checks on you

Your midwife will want to know about your lochia and if you can move your bowels and pee comfortably enough. She will also discuss contraception with you.

Checks on your baby

Newborn babies respond to certain stimuli with reflex actions – such as the grasp reflex, in which a baby will grasp hold of a finger that is brushed against her hand. A paediatrician will test that your baby's baby's reflexes are all present. He or she will also check for physical abnormalities, that the hips are not dislocated and that the heart rate and breathing are normal.

Before you leave

If you have any concerns or questions at all, make sure that you raise these with a midwife before you leave the hospital. If you are not sure how to breastfeed your baby, or bathe her or change her nappy, ask a midwife to show you how. They can also tell you how to take care of the umbilical cord stump.

If you are going home by car, don't forget that your baby needs a car seat!

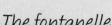

The fontanelle

Two skull bones at the very top of the head of every newborn baby are not joined together to form a hard case, as is the case with the rest of the skull. This is so that the bones can overlap during birth, making it easier for the head to pass down the birth canal. These bones will fuse by the time your baby is a year and a half old. In the meantime, care must be taken with the fontanelle (the name for the soft spot created by the unfused skull bones) so that pressure is not put on the area.

Testing For Abnormalities

Tests can be carried out to discover if your baby has a chromosomal or genetic abnormality. A screening test is first done to determine the risk of your child having an abnormality. Based on these results, you can go on to have a diagnostic test to confirm or rule out an abnormality.

Serum screening tests

All pregnant women are offered a serum screening test which takes place at the end of the first trimester or the start of the second trimester. It involves a blood test to detect certain substances in your blood. It then takes into consideration factors including your age, weight, ethnicity and the gestational age (see page 43) of your baby, to calculate a risk factor for specific abnormalities.

If you decide to have a screening test, remember that it cannot give you a definitive answer on whether or not your baby has an abnormality. It can provide you with the probability of your baby being born with an abnormality. There are four types of screening tests available in the UK.

Types of test

The combined test must be carried out between 11 weeks plus 2 days and 14 weeks plus 1 day of pregnancy. Providing you have your booking appointment early enough for it to be arranged, you'll be offered this test (and if not, you'll be offered the quadruple test or the triple test).

The combined test screens for Down's syndrome, as well as other chromosomal abnormalities. There are two elements to the test (hence the name): a blood test and the nuchal translucency scan (see page 45).

The quadruple test takes place between 14 weeks plus 2 days and 20 weeks precisely. It screens for alpha-fetoprotein beta-hCG, estriol and inhibin A which can give a risk factor for Down's syndrome.

The triple test takes place between 14 weeks plus 2 days and 20 weeks precisely. It screens for serum levels of alphafetoprotein, estriol and beta, hCG giving a risk factor for Down's syndrome. This blood test is less reliable than the combined test.

The Harmony prenatal DNA test is offered by few hospitals on the NHS, but you can have it done privately. By checking traces of the baby's DNA found in the mother's blood, it screens for three chromosomal abnormalities: Down's syndrome, Patau's syndrome and Edwards syndrome. It can be done from 12 weeks of pregnancy. There are two elements involved: a scan and a blood test.

Accuracy of results

Some tests have more accurate results than others, with lower false positives (which is where a positive result is later found out to be wrong). Lower rates of false positive rates are good because a false positive result could result in a mother needlessly taking a diagnostic test (see below), which come with a risk of miscarriage.

The combined test accurately predicts 90 per cent of cases of Down's syndrome, and the false positive rate is 5 per cent. The quadruple test has the same level of accuracy and false positive rate as the combined test. The triple test is less accurate, with a detection rate of approximately 75 per cent, and a 58 per cent false positive rate. The most accurate test is the Harmony test, which is 99 per cent accurate at detecting Down's syndrome,

97 per cent accurate at detecting Edwards syndrome and 80 per cent accurate at detecting Patau's syndrome, with a 0.1 per cent false positive rate. As the triple test is the least accurate, if you are offered only this test by your hospital, consider paying for the others to be conducted privately.

Interpreting the results

Results are usually available within five working days, or two weeks in the case of the Harmony test. Ask your midwife, GP or obstetrician to help you understand the results and their implications. If they suggest that your baby has an abnormality, you will be offered a diagnostic test, and your midwife, GP or obstetrician will advise you further.

Diagnostic tests

There are three diagnostic tests for abnormalities, each of which can confirm for certain whether or not your baby has a specific condition, giving you a chance to prepare for raising a child with a disability, or to terminate the pregnancy. Your midwife, GP or obstetrician will tell you which test is most suitable to your situation.

Each test has a risk of miscarriage, so you must be sure that the risk is something that you are willing to bear. This is an entirely personal choice, and one you may be able to make easily, or you may need time to deliberate. Your healthcare providers can give you guidance, and there are support groups that can help – ask your midwife for information.

Amniocentesis

Chromosomal abnormalities such as Down's syndrome, Patau's syndrome and Edwards syndrome can be detected with an amniocentesis. It is preferable for this test to take place between weeks 14 and 16 of pregnancy, but it can be done up to the end of week 26.

The procedure takes roughly half an hour. Anaesthetic in the form of a gel is applied to the mother's abdomen, and a local anaesthetic may also be injected into the skin. Guided by ultrasound scan, an obstetrician inserts a fine needle through the tummy into the womb, to take some amniotic fluid. Results are available within two weeks – or more quickly if you are able and willing to pay for newer diagnostic techniques. The test comes with a 1 per cent chance of miscarriage. With the most experienced obstetricians, this falls to 0.3 per cent.

Chorionic villus sampling

CVS detects chromosomal or genetic abnormalities. The test may be carried out during weeks 11 to 13 of pregnancy. The procedure is done in the same way as an amniocentesis, but the obstetrician takes a sample of tissue from the placenta. In a few cases, the test is done via the vagina and cervix. Results are usually available within seven days. The test comes with a 1 per cent chance of miscarriage, which falls considerably if the obstetrician who conducts the test is highly experienced.

Cordocentesis

This test detects chromosomal abnormalities. It can be performed after week 18 of pregnancy and is most commonly carried out if amniocentesis or CVS has not provided a reliable diagnosis. It is conducted in the same way as an amniocentesis, but this time a sample of the baby's blood is taken from the umbilical cord. Results are usually available within three days.

Recovering from the test

Get plenty of rest directly after a diagnostic test. You may experience abdominal cramps and light bleeding from the vagina. Most miscarriages after a test are caused by infection, so you'll need to monitor your temperature for a couple of weeks. Contact your obstetrician immediately if your temperature rises above 37.3°C, you experience flu symptoms or feel unwell, or if you think amniotic fluid is leaking (indicated by wet underwear). An infection can be treated with antibiotics.

Miscarriage, Stillbirth and Premature Birth

In very few cases, things go wrong. Your healthcare team will do all they can to take care of you and help you through the experience. There are also support groups that can help.

Miscarriage

Miscarriage is defined as losing a baby before 24 weeks. Many factors can be the cause: infection, maternal age, diabetes, smoking and genetic conditions are common reasons. A weak cervix may cause a miscarriage later in pregnancy. In many cases, it's hard to discover why a miscarriage occurred and difficult to establish why, even by testing, which can be doubly heartbreaking for a mother who needs to know why she lost her baby.

If miscarriage occurs during the first trimester, it is termed an 'early' miscarriage; in the second trimester is known as a 'late' miscarriage. Three or more miscarriages in a row are referred to as recurrent miscarriage.

Early miscarriage

Roughly two-thirds of early miscarriages happen because the baby has a chromosomal disorder that's 'incompatible with life'. If this happens to you, unless both you and your partner are carriers of the same genetic abnormality, it's unlikely this will affect your chances of becoming pregnant again and having a healthy baby in the future.

The experience is much like having a heavy period and, if it takes place towards the end of the first trimester, it might involve abdominal cramps. (In a few instances, there are no symptoms.) An ultrasound scan, conducted at an Early Pregnancy Unit, will confirm whether or not a miscarriage is under way and if, it has taken place, if all the pregnancy tissues are expelled. If the scan confirms the baby has died but is still in the womb, or that some pregnancy tissue remains in the womb, your healthcare team will advise you on what should happen next in your case. In most cases, bleeding happens naturally, but to ensure the womb is clear of tissues (to avoid infection), a course of pills combined with a pessary may be prescribed. In a few cases, tissues are removed surgically.

Late miscarriage

Miscarriages that take place during the second trimester are usually caused by blood disorders, an infection, severe food poisoning or a problem with the umbilical cord, placenta, cervix or womb. As with early miscarriage, bleeding and cramping suggest that a miscarriage is taking place and. During the latter part of the second trimester, the waters may break, too, and there may also be contractions. Alternatively, there may be no symptoms and the loss of the baby's life is detected at a routine ultrasound scan.

Stillbirth and neonatal death

When a baby has died in the womb after 24 weeks of pregnancy, the death is referred to as a stillbirth. If a baby dies within four weeks of birth it is known as a neonatal death. Around 30 per cent of still births are due to the baby being unable to grow in the womb due to intrauterine growth restriction. Chromosomal abnormalities are responsible for roughly 6 per cent of stillbirths. Other causes include diabetes, placental abruptions, maternal infection or pre-eclampsia. Approximately 500 babies per year die in labour. Neonatal death is caused by congenital conditions in 23 per cent of babies. Premature rupture of the membranes, intrauterine growth restriction or lack of oxygen during birth accounts for 20 per cent of neonatal deaths. Neonatal infection causes 13 per cent of neonatal deaths. Other causes include poor placental function, haemorrhage and prematurity.

Delivering the baby

Your obstetrician will explain all the options when it comes to delivering the baby. They'll recommend a vaginal delivery as it creates fewer risks for future deliveries, but if you prefer a Caesarean section, your obstetrician will discuss the risks with you.

A vaginal delivery is usually induced to prevent infections or bleeding. It takes place in a delivery room that is adapted for the delivery of stillborn babies. Your partner will be able to stay with you. A specially trained midwife will help you during the delivery and you'll be offered pain relief. Once delivery has taken place, the staff will give you and your partner privacy with your baby and help you collect any mementos you need, such as a lock of your baby's hair and handprints and footprints.

After the delivery

The hospital staff will talk you through all you need to do to recover from the delivery, and the obstetrician will want to check on your recovery a few weeks after the delivery. Staff will help you if you wish to find out what was the cause of death.

Losing a baby

Losing your baby is one of the most difficult things for a parent to go through. You and your partner must give yourselves space and time to grieve for your child – and get as much help through the experience as possible. Your midwife will be able to provide you with a list of organisations that support parents who have gone through miscarriage, stillbirth or neonatal death.

Premature birth

A birth that takes place before 37 weeks is referred to as a 'premature' birth. It stands to reason that a baby born closer to the due date has a better chance of survival than one born much before the due date. For example, a baby born at 26 weeks has a 78 per cent chance of survival, which drops to 42 per cent at 24 weeks. Survival of a baby born at 23 weeks is rare. Babies born very early have a higher chance of having an abnormality.

The cause of premature birth in 40 per cent of cases is unexplained. A likely cause is maternal infection. About 20 per cent of cases happen due to premature rupture of the membranes. In 25 per cent of cases, a medical condition, such as diabetes, placental abruption, placenta praevia, placental insufficiency, fetal abnormality or fetal growth restriction is the cause. If you have had a previous premature delivery, your healthcare team will keep a close eye on you throughout pregnancy to try to avoid the same thing happening again.

Onset of labour

If your waters break, you begin to feel contractions, or you experience a show (see page 104), contact your midwife immediately, who will arrange a test to check if labour has begun. Your obstetrician will advise you according to which week of pregnancy you are in and if your waters have broken or your contractions have begun (both of which require a different approach). The team will try to keep the baby in the womb for as long as possible, to give you steroids that help to speed up maturation of her lungs and give her the best chance of survival. Drugs can slow down and stop contractions if necessary and viable. If labour can't be stopped, you may deliver vaginally or by Caesarean section. After delivery, your baby will be taken to a neonatal unit, where the staff are trained to help unwell newborns and premature babies. You will be able to join her when you have recovered from the birth.

Index

Editorial Director Anne Furniss
Creative Director Helen Lewis
Project Editor Victoria Marshallsay
Reasearch and Text Salima Hirani
Design Katherine Keeble
Design Assistant Emily Lapworth
Illustrations Annamaria Dutto
Photography Tiffany Mumford
Production Director Vincent Smith
Production Controller Sasha Hawkes

Many thanks to the parents and babies who kindly allowed themselves to be photographed for this book.

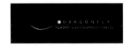 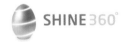

British Library Cataloguing-in-Publication Data. A catalogue record of this book is available from the British Library.

ISBN: 978 184949 560 8

Printed in China